BIOCHEMISTRY
AND
CLINICAL PATHOLOGY

(THEORY AND PRACTICAL)

BIOCHEMISTRY
AND
CLINICAL PATHOLOGY

(THEORY AND PRACTICAL)

By

K.K. PILLAI
M.Pharm., Ph.D.
Reader in Pharmacology
Faculty of Pharmacy, Jamia Hamdard
Hamdard Nagar, New Delhi-110062

and

J.S. QADRY
M. Pharm. (Pb), D.Sc. (Münster),
M.S.E.I., F.G.F.A. (Tubingen)
Professor of Pharmacognosy
Faculty of Pharmacy, Jamia Hamdard
Hamdard Nagar, New Delhi-110062

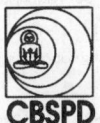

CBSPD

CBS Publishers & Distributors Pvt Ltd

New Delhi • Bengaluru • Chennai • Kochi • Kolkata • Lucknow • Mumbai
Gujarat • Hyderabad • Jharkhand • Nagpur • Patna • Pune • Uttarakhand

Biochemistry and Clinical Pathology
(Theory and Practical)

ISBN: 978-81-239-0289-0

© Publisher

First Edition: 1994
Reprint: 1998, 2001,2002, 2004, 2005, 2007, 2008, 2010, 2012, 2015, 2017, 2018, 2019, 2021, 2024, **2026**

Published by **Satish Kumar** Jain and Produced by **Varun Jain** for

CBS Publishers & Distributors Pvt Ltd

4819/XI Prahlad Street, 24 Ansari Road, Daryaganj, New Delhi 110 002, India.

Ph: 011-23289259, 23266861, 23266867
Fax: 011-23243014

Website: www.cbspd.com
e-mail: delhi@cbspd.com;
cbspubs@airtelmail.in.

Corporate Office: 204 FIE, Industrial Area, Patparganj, Delhi 110 092, India
Ph: 011-4934 4934
Fax: 011-4934 4935

e-mail: publishing@cbspd.com;
publicity@cbspd.com

Branches

- **Bengaluru:** Seema House 2975, 17th Cross, KR Road, Banasankari 2nd Stage, Bengaluru 560 070, Karnataka, India
  Ph: +91-80-26771678/79   Fax: +91-80-26771680   e-mail: bangalore@cbspd.com
- **Chennai:** 18/8B, Subbaraya Street, Shenoy Nagar, Chennai 600 030, Tamil Nadu, India
  Ph: +91-044-42032115, 044-26681266   e-mail: chennai@cbspd.com
- **Kochi:** 42/1325, 1326, Power House Road, Opp KSEB, Power House, Ernakulum Kochi 682 018, Kerala, India
  Ph: +91-484-4059061-65,67   Fax: +91-484-4059065   e-mail: kochi@cbspd.com
- **Kolkata:** 147, Hind Ceramics Compound, 1st Floor, Nilgunj Road, Belghoria, Kolkata-700056, West Bengal, India
  Ph: +033-25633055, 033-25633056   e-mail: kolkata@cbspd.com
- **Lucknow:** Basement, Khushnuma Complex, 7 Meerabai Marg (Behind Jawahar Bhawan), Lucknow-226001, UP, India
  Ph: +0522-4000032   e-mail: tiwari.lucknow@cbspd.com
- **Mumbai:** PWD Shed, Gala no 25/26, Ramchandra Bhatt Marg, Next to JJ Hospital Gate no. 2, Opp. Union Bank of India, Noorbaug, Mumbai-400009, Maharashtra, India
  Ph: 022-66661880/89   e-mail: mumbai@cbspd.com

Representatives

• Gujarat	0-9879558667	• Hyderabad	0-9885175004	• Jharkhand	0-9811541605
• Nagpur	0-8692091830	• Patna	0-9334159340	• Pune	0-9664372571
• Uttarakhand	0-9716462459				

Printed at SRK Graphics, Delhi (India)

PREFACE

We have written this book with the needs of Diploma in Pharmacy students as per the new Education Regulation in our minds. We hope that this book may also be useful as a quick reference book for degree students. We have dealt with the theory as well as the practical in the same book. The subject of biochemistry has assumed importance in the Diploma in Pharmacy course only after the implementation of new Education Regulation in Pharmacy Institutions in this country. Knowledge of biochemistry is very essential to understand the emerging trends in Pharmaceutical sciences. We are grateful to Mr. Satish Kumar Jain, Managing Director, CBS Publishers and Distributors for the encouragement and suggestions and we are thankful to Mr. Sunil Kumar Dhir for best laser typesetting of this book. We would like to thank Mr. Zakir Husain, Head, Department of Pharmacology, Jamia Hamdard, for his advice. Many thanks are extended to Mr. B.R. Sharma, Mr. Jitinder and other staff of CBS Publishers for expedicting the production of this book. We thank profusely our family members, who helped us in every possible way. We shall welcome constructive suggestions.

K.K. PILLAI

J.S. QADRY

CONTENTS

BIOCHEMISTRY PRACTICAL

Section - I

Section - II

1

INTRODUCTION

Biochemistry is the science which deals with the chemistry of living tissues and the substances that take part in their metabolism. Optimal level of biochemicals in a living organism keep the organism in healthy condition. Either excess or low concentration of biochemicals will affect the function of a living organism which leads to a disease state. Therefore, understanding of biochemistry is very useful in the diagnosis and treatment of various diseases.

Biochemistry in preventive medicine

Knowledge of biochemistry can be utilized to prevent malnutrition. Similarly estimations of biochemicals like blood cholesterol, or enzymes can help the clinicians to find atherosclerosis or cancer at an early stage. Thus, doctors can advise the patients to take preventive steps according to the nature of the disease.

Many genetic disorders like phenylketonuria, glucose-6-phosphate dehydrogenase deficiency can be identified by the use of clinical biochemistry.

Knowledge of biochemistry is very essential for designing many drugs useful in variety of pathological conditions. A sound knowledge of biochemistry is required to understand the metabolism of drugs by different enzymes. Toxic substances act on biochemical reactions or processes in the living cells, thus study of toxicology also requires a better understanding of biochemistry. Advances in nuclear biochemistry is useful in the field of recombiant DNA technology to synthesize many bioactive polypeptide like human insulin.

2

PROTEINS

Proteins are complex nitrogenous substance of high molecular weight which on decomposition by acids, alkalis or enzymes yield aminoacids.

Proteins play a vital role in our body. Following are some of the chief function of the proteins in our body.

(i) Protein is a part of the cell membrane structure.

(ii) Structural proteins are present in different organs of our body.

(iii) All enzymes are proteins

(iv) Contractile proteins. like actin myosin and others are essential for muscular contraction.

(v) Many clotting factors are proteins.

(vi) Immunoglobulins are proteins in nature.

(vii) Conjugate protein-like hemoglobin is very essential for oxygentransport from blood into the cells.

(viii) Many hormones are polypeptides in nature (e.g. Insulin, Parathormone).

Peptide bonds

Peptide bonds, Unite the amino end (N-terminal) of one amino acid to the carboxyl end (C-terminal) of another.

$$H_2N - \overset{\overset{\displaystyle R_1}{|}}{CH} - COOH + H_2N - \overset{\overset{\displaystyle R_2}{|}}{CH} - COOH$$

$$\downarrow H_2O$$

$$H_2N - \overset{\overset{\displaystyle R_1}{|}}{CH} - \overset{\overset{\displaystyle O}{\|}}{C} - NH - \overset{\overset{\displaystyle R_2}{|}}{CH} - COOH$$

Peptide bond

Each aminoacid in a polypeptide chain is termed a residue.

Oligopeptide : An amino acid chain with less than 25 amino acid is called an oligopeptide.

e.g. TRH (Thyrotrophin releasing hormone)

Enkephalins	Motilin
Angiotensin II	Gastrin
Vasopressin	Substance P
Oxytocin	Somatostatin
Bradykinin	Bombesin
Glucagon	Endothelin

Polypeptide : An amino acid chain with more than 25 amino acids is called a polypeptide.

e.g. Insulin
VIP (Vasoactive intestinal peptide)
ACTH (Adreno corticotrophic hormone)
Neuropeptide Y

Protein : A protein may consist of a long polypeptide chain or several polypeptide subunits.

e.g. Streptokinase
Tissue plasminogen activator
Interferons
Clotting factors
Antibodies

Determination of primary structure of protein

It involves two steps :

(a) Qualitative identification and quantitative estimation of aminoacid residue.

(b) Determination of linear order or sequence:peptide bond hydrolysis or proteolysis is done by proteolytic enzymes, acids or alkali and the free amino acids are separated by chromatography.

Acid hydrolysis of protein

$$\text{Protein} \xrightarrow[\text{at } 110^{\circ}\text{C for 24 hrs.}]{6 \text{ NHCl}} \text{Aminoacids}$$

Set back of acid hydrolysis

Amino acids like tryptophan and cysteine are destroyed where as serine, threonine and tyrosine are partially destroyed.

Hydrolysis of protein by alkali

Alkaline hydrolysis does not damage tryptophan, hence, alkaline hydrolysis can be used to separate tryptophan from peptides. However, alkaline hydrolysis destroys cysteine, serine, and threonine.

Hydrolysis of protein by enzymes

Enzymes catalysed hydrolysis depends upon the nature of the enzymes

e.g. Peptidase hydrolyses all proteins but very slowly.

Chymotrypsin : Attacks peptide bond at the carboxyl side of tyrosine and phenylalanine.

Pepsin : Attacks peptide bond at the amino side of tyrosine and phenylalanine.

Trypsin : Hydrolyses the peptide bond at the carboxyl side of lysine and arginine

Carboxypeptidase

It splits peptide bonds adjacent to a free carboxyl group. As soon as the first amino acid is split from the chain the enzyme attacks the second peptide bond of the polypeptide. The residue bearing the free aminogroup of peptide chain is called as N-terminal residue and the one bearing the α-carboxyl group is called as C-terminal residue.

$$H_2N - CH - C {\overset{O}{\underset{\parallel}{\|}}} NH - CH - C - NH - CH - C {\|} NH - CH - C {\|} NH - CH$$

with side chains CH_2, CH_2, CH_2, CH_2—NH_2 (Lysine); R, O; R_1; CH_2 (with OH phenyl, Tyrosine), O; R_3

Trypsin   Pepsin   Chymotrypsin

Lysine   Tyrosine

N-terminal   Dipeptide   C-terminal

$$H_2N - CH - C - HN - CH - COOH$$
$$\quad\quad CH_3 \;\; O \quad\quad CH_2 - OH$$

Ala   Ser
(Alanine)   (Serine)

Determination of N-terminal aminoacid residue

In 1945 Sanger introduced the use of 1-fluoro-2, 4 dinitrobenzene to determine the N-terminal aminoacid residue.

$$O_2N - \langle \rangle - F + H - N(H) - CH - COOH \xrightarrow{HF} O_2N - \langle \rangle - NH \, CH - COOh$$
with NO_2 and R groups

1-fluoro-2, 4 dinitrobenzene   Nitrophenyl peptide
DNFB

OR.

$$O_2N - \langle \rangle - NH - CH - CO - NH - CH - CO - NH - CH - CO - NH - CH - COOH$$
with NO_2 and R, R_1, R_2, R_3 groups

α-aminogroup of peptide reacts with DNFB to form a yellow 2, 4 dinitrophenyl derivative when this derivative is subjected to acid hydrolysis by 6NHCl all the peptide bonds are hydrolysed except the bond between DNFB and N-terminal aminoacid which is more stable to acid hydrolysis.

This nitrophenyl derivative is separated from free aminoacid, identified and compared with standard dinitrophenyl derivative.

Fluorimetric method for determination of N-terminal amino acid

Dansylchloride

1-dimethylaminonaphthalene

5-sulfonylchloride

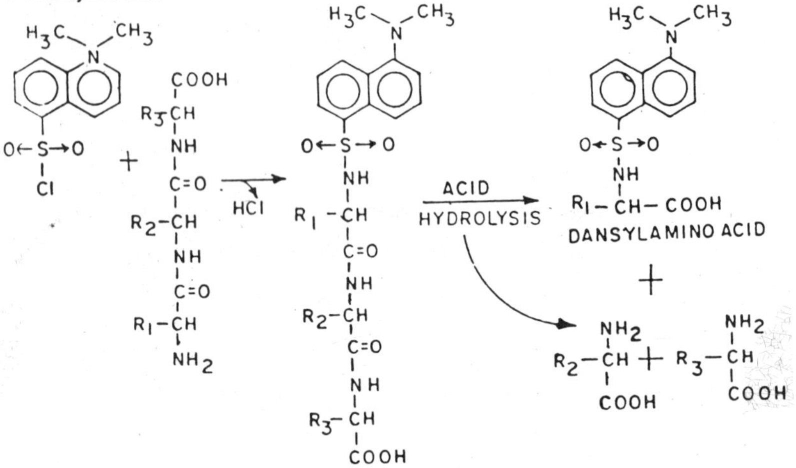

DANSYLTRIPEPTIDE

Dansylaminoacid is measured by fluorimetric method (This method is 100 times more sensitive than the DNFB method).

Identification of N-terminal residue by the Edman degradation.

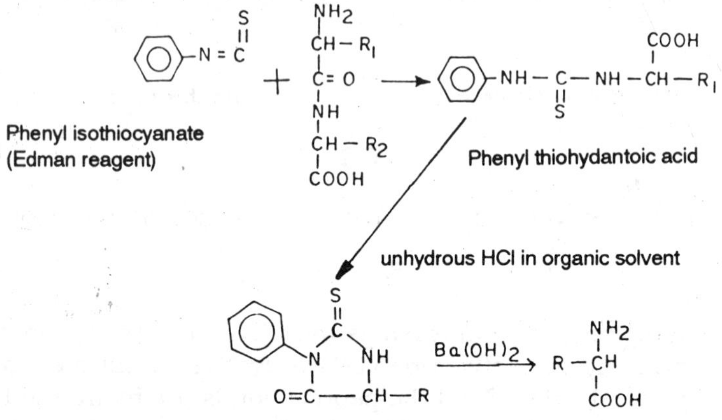

Phenyl isothiocyanate (Edman reagent)

Phenyl thiohydantoic acid

unhydrous HCl in organic solvent

Phenylthio hydantoin

Phenylthiohydantoin is soluble in organic solvent and is determined by gas liquid chromatography.

Determination of C-terminal residue

The C-terminal residue can be identified by using hydrazine. Hydrazine reacts with peptide and forms aminoacylhydrazine which can be determined by chromatography.

Carboxypeptidase enzyme is also used to find out C-terminal amino acid. Carboxypeptidase attacks C-terminal peptide bond of a protein.

CLASSIFICATION OF PROTEINS

I. Simple Protein

These proteins on hydrolysis yield amino acids.

e.g. Albumin
Globulin
Prolamine
Glutelins
Scleroprotein

II. Conjugated protein

These proteins on hydrolysis yield amino acid and a prosthetic group.

Class	Prosthetic group
(a) Nucleoprotein	Ribonucleic acid Deoxy ribonucleic acid
(b) Lipoprotein	Phospholipid Cholesterol Neutral lipid
(c) Glycoproteins	Hexosamine, galactose Mannose, Sialic acid
(d) Phosphoprotein Casein	Phosphate esterified with serine
(e) Hemoproteins Hemoglobin Cytochrome Catalase	Iron protoporphyrin

Class	Prosthetic group
(f) Flavoproteins Succinic acid dehydrogenase D-amino acid oxidase	FAD
(g) Metalloproteins Ferritin Cytochrome oxidase Alcoholdehydrogenase Xanthine oxidase	Fe Fe and Cu Zn Mo

Classification of protein based upon biological function

Types and Examples	Function
I. Enzymes	
Hexokinase	Phosphorylation
Cytochrome C	Transfer of electron
DNA polymerase	Replication and repair of DNA
II. Storage proteins	
Ova albumin	Egg white protein
Casein	Milk protein
Ferritin	Iron storage protein
III. Transport protein	
Hemoglobin	Transport of oxygen in blood of vertebrates
Hemocyanin	Transport of oxygen in blood of in-vertebrate
Myoglobin	Transport of oxygen in muscle cells
Lipoproteins	Transport of lipid in blood
Iron binding globulin	Transport of iron in blood
Ceruloplasmin	Transport of Cu ++ in blood

Types and Examples	Function
IV. Contractile proteins	
Actin	Contraction of muscles.
Myosin	
V. Protective proteins	
Antibodies	Form complex with foreign protein
Complement	Form complex with antigen antibody
Fibrinogen	Precursor of fibrin
Thrombin	Component of clotting mechanism
VI. Toxins	
Clostridium botulinumtoxin	Protein causing food poisoning
VII. Hormones	
Insulin	Regulates blood sugar
VIII. Structural protein	
α-keratin	Skin
Collagen	Fibrous connective tissue.

All living organisms contain α-amino acids and all aminoacids share the same structural backbone.

$$
\begin{array}{l}
\text{NH}_2 \quad\quad \alpha\text{-amino group} \\
| \\
\text{R} - \text{C} - \text{H} \quad \alpha\text{-carbonatom} \\
| \\
\text{C} = \text{O} \quad\quad \alpha\text{-carboxyl group} \\
| \\
\text{OH}
\end{array}
$$

All α-aminoacids have three main features

1. They have an α-amino group

2. They possess a side chain, or R group, that is bound to that α-carbonatom.

3. They contain an α-carboxyl group.

Classification of amino acid : About twenty amino acids are generally found in most proteins

I. Aminoacids with aliphatic side chain (Neutral amino acids)

1. Glycine   Gly   Aminoacetic acid

$$H—CH—COOH$$
$$\quad\quad |$$
$$\quad\quad NH_2$$

2. Alanine   Ala α-aminopropionic acid

$$CH_3—CH—COOH$$
$$\quad\quad\quad |$$
$$\quad\quad\quad NH_2$$

3. Valine   Val α-aminoisovaleric acid

$$CH_3 \quad CH_3$$
$$\diagdown \diagup$$
$$CH\text{-}COOH$$
$$\quad |$$
$$\quad NH_2$$

4. Leucine   Leu α-aminoisocaproic acid

$$CH_3$$
$$\quad\diagdown$$
$$\quad\quad CH—CH_2—CH—COOH$$
$$\quad\diagup \quad\quad\quad\quad\quad |$$
$$CH_3 \quad\quad\quad\quad\quad NH_2$$

5. Isoleucine Ileu α-amino β-methyl valeric acid

$$CH_3$$
$$|$$
$$CH_2$$
$$\quad\diagdown$$
$$\quad\quad CH\text{-}CH\text{-}COOH$$
$$\quad\diagup \quad\quad\quad |$$
$$CH_3 \quad\quad NH_2$$

II. Hydroxylsubstituted amino acids (Neutral amino acids)

1. Serine Ser α-amino β-hydroxy propionic acid

$$CH_2—CH—COOH$$
$$\;|\quad\quad |$$
$$OH\quad NH_2$$

2. Threonine Thr. α-amino β-hydroxy   n-butyric acid

$$CH_3—CH—CH—COOH$$
$$OH \quad NH_2$$

Threonine

III. Sulphur containing amino acids

1. Cysteine cys   α-amino β-mercapto propionic acid

$$HS—CH_2—CH—COOH$$
$$NH_2$$

2. Cystine cys-s-s-cys β, β, dithio α-amino   propionic acid

$$HOOC—CH—CH_2—S—S—CH_2—CH—COOH$$
$$NH_2 NH_2$$

3. Methionine Met   α-amino-γ-methylthio n-butyric acid

$$CH_2—CH_2—CH—COOH$$
$$S—CH_3 NH_2$$

IV. Aromatic amino acids derived from alanine

1. Phenylalanine Phe   α-amino β-phenyl propionic acid

$$\bigcirc\!-CH_2 - CH - COOH$$
$$NH_2$$

2. Tyrosine   Tyr   α-amino β (p-hydroxyphenyl) propionic acid

$$HO-\bigcirc\!-CH_2 - CH - COOH$$
$$NH_2$$

3. Tryoptophan   Trp.   α-amino β-indole propionic acid

$$-CH_2—CH—COOH$$
$$NH_2$$

V. Acidic aminoacids

1. Aspartic acid Asp   α-amino succinic acid

$$HOOCCH_2 - CH - COOH$$
$$NH_2$$

2. Asparagine   Asn   γ-amide of α-amino succinic acid

$$O$$
$$H_2N - C - CH_2CHCOOH$$
$$NH_2$$

3. Glutamic acid Glu   α-aminoglutaric acid

$$HOOC—CH_2—CH_2—\underset{\underset{NH_2}{|}}{CH}—COOH$$

4. Glutamine Gln   δ-amide of α-amino glutaric acid

$$H_2N—\overset{\overset{O}{||}}{C}—CH_2—CH_2—\underset{\underset{NH_2}{|}}{CH}—COOH$$

VI. Basic amino acid

1. Arginine Arg. α-amino δ-guanidino n-valeric acid

$$NH—CH_2—CH_2—CH_2—\underset{\underset{NH_2}{|}}{CH}—COOH$$
$$\underset{\underset{NH_2}{|}}{C}{=}NH$$

2. Lysine Lys   α, ε- diamino caproic acid

$$\underset{\underset{NH_2}{|}}{CH_2}—CH_2—CH_2—CH_2—\underset{\underset{NH_2}{|}}{CH}—COOH$$

3. Histidine His   α-amino β-imidazole Propionic acid

$$CH_2—\underset{\underset{NH_2}{|}}{CH}—COOH$$

VII. Imino acids

1. Proline Pro   Pyrrolidine 2-carboxylic acid

COOH

2. 4-hydroxyproline Hyp   4-Hydroxypyrrolidine
                          2 -carboxylic acid

COOH

Except glycine, all other amino acids are optically active compounds, and those found in naturally occuring proteins are all L-amino acids.

QUALITATIVE TESTS FOR PROTEINS

Biuret test

To 2-3 ml of protein solution in a test tube add an equal volume of 10% sodium hydroxide solution, Mix thoroughly and add a 0.5% coppersulphate solution drop by drop until a purplish violet colour is produced. Biuret test is positive for those molecules which contain two carbamyl group (Co-NH₂) joined either directly together or through a single atom of nitrogen or carbon.

Ninhydrin reaction

To 5 ml of dilute protein solution (pH between 5 and 7) add 0.5 ml of a 0.1% solution of ninhydrin. Heat to boiling for 2 minutes and allow to cool. Blue colour indicate the presence of protein.

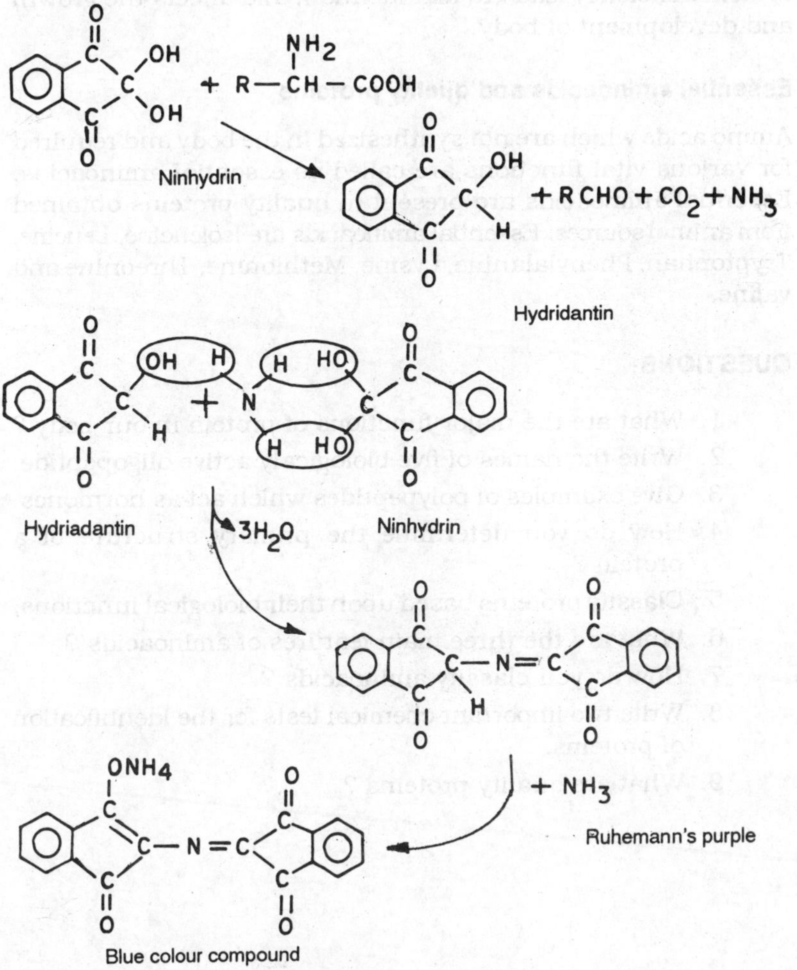

Ninhydrin

Hydridantin

Hydriadantin   3H₂O   Ninhydrin

Ruhemann's purple

Blue colour compound

The ninhydrin reaction can be used to estimate the quantity of amino acid present in the sample. Individual amino acids can be separated by chromatoraphic techniques for estimation.

Biological value

Amino acids are very essential for the biosynthesis of enzymes, storage proteins, hemoglobin, actin myosin, antibodies, clotting factors and hormones.

Deficiency diseases

Protein deficiency leads to malnutrition, and affects the growth and development of body.

Essential aminoacids and quality proteins

Amino acids which are not synthesized in the body and required for various vital functions are called as essential aminoacids. Essential aminoacids are present in quality proteins obtained from animal sources. Essential aminoacids are Isoleucine, Leucine, Tryptophan, Phenylalanine, Lysine, Methionine, Threonine and valine.

QUESTIONS

1. What are the major functions of protein in our body ?
2. Write the names of five biologicaly active oligopeptide.
3. Give examples of polypeptides which act as hormones.
4. How do you determine the primary structure of a protein ?
5. Classify proteins based upon their biological functions.
6. What are the three main features of aminoacids ?
7. How do you classify aminoacids ?
8. Write two important chemical tests for the identification of proteins.
9. What are quality proteins ?

3

CARBOHYDRATES

Carbohydrates are polyhydroxy aldehydes or ketones or their condensation products. They are important constituent of diet. They are important fuels from which cell derives energy. They are essential to from structural unit of cell membrane complex lipids and proteins. The aldehyde sugars are called aldoses, while with a ketone group are ketoses.

CLASSIFICATION OF CARBOHYDRATES

A. Monosaccharides (Simple sugars)

These are carbohydrates which cannot be hydrolyzed into a simpler form.

1. Trioses
   (a) Aldotriose (e.g. Glyceraldehyde)
   (b) Ketotriose (e.g. Dihydroxyacetone)
2. Tetroses
   (a) Aldosugar (e.g. Erythrose)
   (b) Ketosugar (e.g. Erythrulose)
3. Pentoses
   (a) Aldopentose (e.g. Ribose)
   (b) Ketopentose (e.g. Ribulose)
4. Hexoses
   (a) Aldohexoses (e.g. Glucose, Mannose, galactose)
   (b) Ketohexose (e.g. Fructose)

B. Disaccharides

These are carbohydrates which yield two molecules of same or different monosaccharides on hydrolysis.

(a) Reducing disaccharide e.g. lactose, Maltose

(b) Non-reducing disaccharide e.g. Sucrose

C. Oligosaccharides

On hydrolysis oligosaccharides yield 3-6 monosaccharide units.

e.g.   Maltotriose

D. Polysaccharides

These carbohydrates on hydrolysis yield more than 6 monosaccharide units.

1. Homopolysaccharides e.g. Starch, glycogen
2. Heteropolysaccharides e.g. Heparin, Hyaluronic acid.

Monosaccharides exhibit isomerism,

          D-Glyceraldehyde   L-Glyceraldehyde

D and L indicate spatial relationship and not optical activity. Optical activity is denoted by + (d-form) and - (l-form).

When two mono saccharide units condense together with elimination of water a disaccharide is formed.

Mutarotation

When glucose is dissolved in water, the solution has specific rotation of a D + 111°, when the solution is allowed to stand rotation falls slowly ot 52.5 Similarly β-glucose gives rotation from 19° to 52°.

It indicates that glucose can exist in two forms. The change in rotation to a common value which occurs when either of this two form is allowed to stand in solution is known as Mutarotation.

The configuration of C-atom 1 of glucose is denoted either by α or β form. If C-1 OH is on right side it is α form and if it is on left side it is β - form.

α-D-glucose   β–D-glucose

Glucose is the carbohydrate utilised by cells. Galactose & fructose are converted to glucose for utilization. In the body glucose is stored in the form of glycogen and is stored in liver. Blood contains 60-90mg of glucose per 100 ml. In diabetes the fasting sugar level is more than 120 mg/100 ml.

Reactions of glucose

(a) Glucose is a reducing agent. So capable of reducing cupric compound to cuprous state

$$\text{Glucose} + \text{CuSO}_4 \xrightarrow[\text{Sodiumcitrate}]{\text{Na}_2\text{CO}_3} \underset{\substack{\text{Yellow or} \\ \text{red precipitate}}}{\text{Cu}_2\text{O}}$$

The above property of glucose is used in estimating glucose in biological fluids

(b) $\text{Glucose} \xrightarrow{\text{yeast}} \text{Alcohol} + \text{Co}_2$

(c) **Reactions of alcohol group of glucose :** Glucose readily form esters with phosphoric acid. These phosphoric esters of carbohydrate are very important in the metabolism of carbohydrates.

α-D-glucose 1-phosphate   Glucose - 6- phosphate

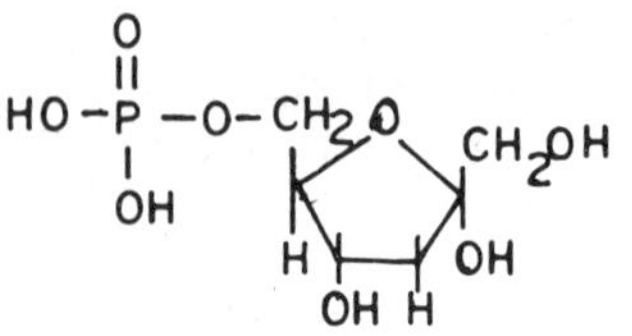

α D Fructose
6-phosphate

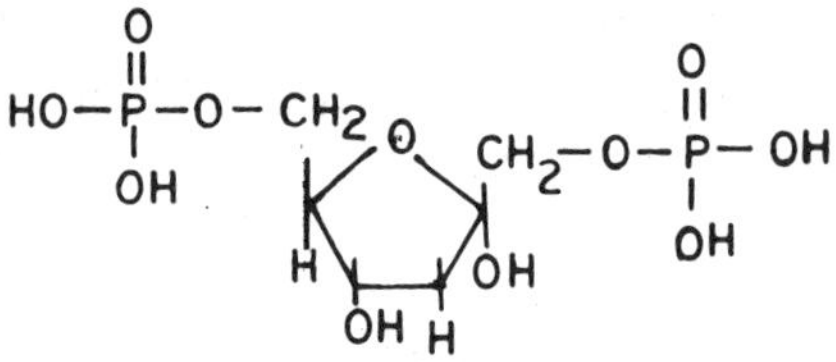

α-D Fructose
1, 6 diphosphate

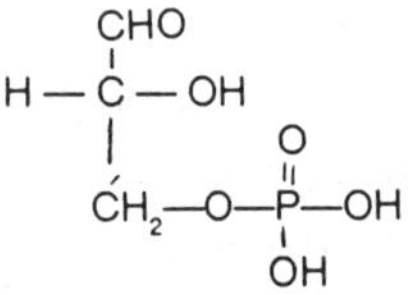

D-glyceraldehyde
3-phosphate

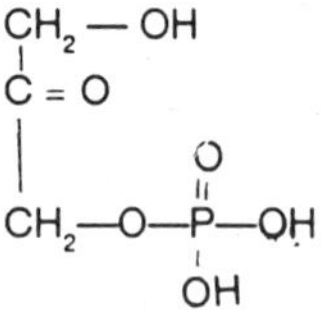

Dihydroxy acetone
3-phosphate

Ribose-5-phosphate is present in RNA• Deoxyribose 5-phosphate is present in DNA.

Reaction with phenylhydrazine

This reaction involves only the carbonylcarbon and the next adjacent carbon. First one mole of carbohydrate and one molecule of phenylhydrazine react to form hydrazones.

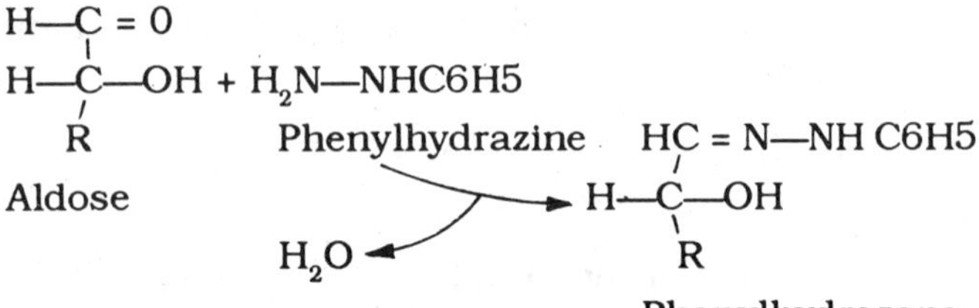

Phenylhydrazone reacts with two additional molecules of phenylhydrazine and forms osazone. These osazones are insoluble in water. They differ in melting point and crystalline structure e.g. Glucosazone, Lactosazone, Maltosazone.

Disaccharides

Disaccharides consist of two monosaccharides joined by a glycosidic bond. The glycosidic bond of disaccharide is classified as α or β and is numbered according to the positions of the carbon atoms it unites.

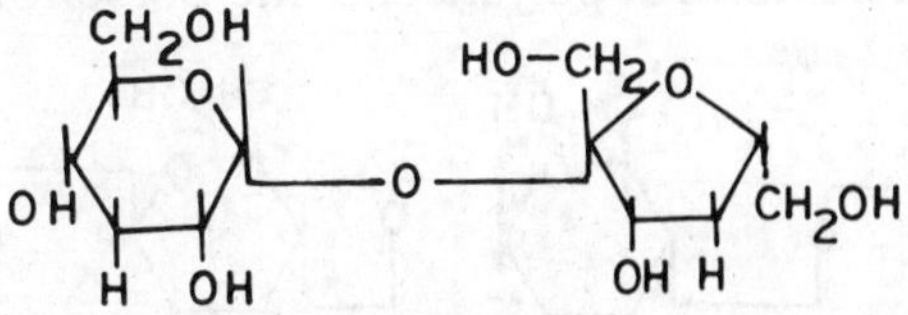

Glucose

Fructose

(α-D-Glucopyranosyl-β-D-fructofuranoside)

Sucrose

Sugars which differ from one another only in the configuration around the reducing carbon are called Anomers. In sucrose, the α-anomeric carbon 1 of glucose joins the β-anomeric carbon 2 of fructose.

Maltose contains two molecules of glucose joined by an α-1, 4 glycosidic bond. It is produced when starch is degraded by the action of amylase during seed germination. Maltose is also produced during gastrointestinal starch digestion.

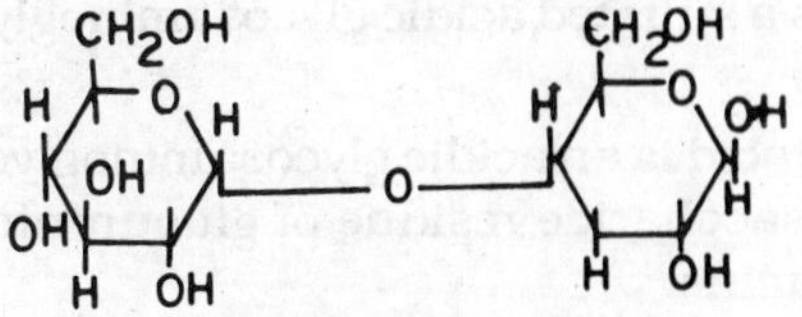

(4-O-α-D-Glucopyranosyl β-D-glucopyranose)

Maltose (β-form)

Lactose is the sugar found in milk. It consists of of β-galactose with a β-1, 4 linkage to glucose.

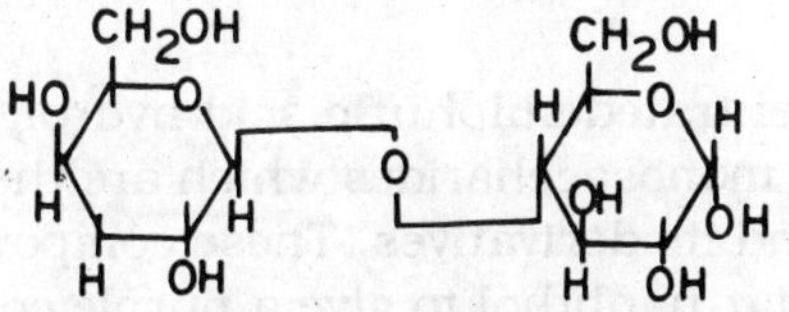

(4-O-β-D-Galactopyranosyl α-D-glucopyranose)

Lactose

Sucrase, maltase and lactase are intestinal enzymes which converts these disaccharide to monosaccharides. Lactase deficiency causes osmotic diarrhoea due to the pesence of undigested lactose in the intestine.

Polysaccharides

Cellulose is a structural polysaccharide present in plants

Glucose β-1, 4 linkage

Cellulose Units

Starch is the energy storing polysaccharide of plants. It contains amylose and amylopectin.

Amylose is a long, unbranched glucose polymer with α-1, 4 bonds. Amylopectin, on the other hand, has α-1, 6 branch linkages spaced about every 30 glucose molecules in its α-1, 4 chain.

Glycogen is the predominant polysaccharide present in the liver of animals. It resembles amylopectin , however, is more highly branched, with α-1, 6 linkages around every 10 glucose units. Heparin is a sulfated acidic glycosaminoglycan present in mast cells.

Hyaluronic acid is an acidic glycosaminoglycan made up of the repeating disaccharide residue of glucuronic acid joined to N-acetylglucosamine.

Qualitative tests for carbohydrates

A 1% solution can be used to carry out the tests

1. Molisch's test

Principle : Concentrated sulphuric acid hydrolyses glycosidic bonds to give the monosaccharides which are then dehydrated to give furfural and its derivatives. These compounds combine with sulphonated α-naphthol to give a purple complex.

Method : Add 2 drops of molisch reagent (5% α-naphthol in ethanol) to 2 ml of test solution and carefully pour about 1 ml of concentrated sulphuric along the side *of the* tube so as to form a layer below the mixture. A red-violet ring appears which indicates the presence of carbohydrates.

2. Iodine test

Iodine forms coloured adsorption complexes with polysaccharides.

Method : Acidify the test solution with dilute hydrochloric acid then add 2 drops of iodine solution and compare the colour with that of water and iodine.

      Starch gives blue colour

      Glycogen gives red colour

      Sugars do not give colour.

3. Barfoed's test

Principle : Barfoed's reagent is weakly acidic and is only reduced by monosaccharides. A precipitate of cuprous oxide is formed. Prolonged boiling may hydrolyse disaccharides to give a false positive reaction.

Method : Add 1 ml of test solution to 2 ml of Barfoed's reagent, boil for one minute in a water bath and observe the colour change after five minutes. If brick-red precipitate occurs with in 5 minutes then the test compound is a monosaccharide and if it becomes brick-red after 7 minutes, it is a disaccharide.

4. Bial's test

Principle : When pentoses are heated with concentrated hydrochloric acid, furfural is formed which condenses orcinol in the presence of ferric ions to give a green colour.

Method : Add 2 ml of test solution to 5 ml of Bial's orcinol solution and heat in a boiling water bath for a few minutes. A green colour indicates the presence of pentoses.

5. Seliwanoff's test

Principle : Ketoses are dehydrated more rapidly than aldoses to give furfural derivative, which condense with resorcinol to form a red complex.

Method : To 1 ml of sample solution add 5 ml of freshly prepared seliwanfoff's reagent and warm in a boiling water bath for Iminute Appearance of cherry red colour indicates the presence of ketoses.

6. Benedicts test

Add 5 drops of test solution to 2 ml of Benedict's reagent and place in a boiling water bath for 5 minutes. A green or yellow or orange red colour indicates the presence of reducing sugars.

Diseases related to carbohydrate metabolism

Diabetes mellitus occurs due to deficiency of insulin. Disturbances in the carbohydrate metabolism also produce ketosis.

QUESTIONS

1. Define the term carbohydrate.
2. Classify carbohydrate with suitable examples.
3. What is meant by mutarotation ?
4. What is the predominant polysaccharide present in the liver ?
5. How do you identify a carbohydrate ?
6. What is meant by diabetesmellitus ?

4

LIPIDS

Lipids are heterogenous group of compound related to fatty acids. (e.g., fats, oils, wax etc.) Lipids are insoluble in water and soluble in organic solvents like ether, chloroform and benzene.

Biological Functions

Lipids form important component of the diet. Lipids act as insulating material in subcutaneous tissue. Lipids also form the structural component of cell membrane and nerve tissue.

CLASSIFICATION

A. Simple lipids

They are esters of fatty acid with various alcohol

Fats : They are esters of fatty acid with glycerol

Waxes : They are esters of fatty acid with higher alcohols.

B. Compound lipids

These are esters of fatty acid containing groups in addition to an alcohol.

Phospholipids : It contains glycerol, fatty acid, phosphate and a nitrogen base. Phospholipids play an important role in the transport of substances in and out of the cells. They are also present in mitochondria, microsomes and nuclei. They insulate enzymes in the mitochondria. They are many types of phospholipid.

e.g.   Lecithins
        Cephalins
        Phosphatidylserine
        Phosphoinositides
        Plasmalogens
        Phosphatidicacid
        Sphingomyelins
        Lysophospholipids

Glycolipids

It contains fatty acid, sphingosine and a carbohydrate.

e.g.   Cerebrosides

C. Derived Lipids

e.g.   Glycerol,
        Fatty acids,
        Cholesterol,
        Steroid

Fatty acids

Fatty acids are obtained by the hydrolysis of fats. They may be either saturated or unsaturated fatty acids.

Saturated fatty acids

e.g.   Acetic acid
        Butyric acid
        Palmitic acid
        Stearic acid etc.

Unsaturated fatty acids

They are also called essential fatty acids.

e.g.   Oleic acid
        Linoleic acid
        Linolenic acid

All fatty acids have a single COOH groups at the end of a hydrocarbon chain·Fatty acids are weak acids. Acetic acid is the simplest fatty acid.

FATTY ACIDS FOUND IN NATURAL FATS

Saturated fatty acids		Source
Butyric acid	$CH_3 (CH_2)_2 COOH$	Milk, Butter
Caproic acid	$CH_3 (CH_2)_4 COOH$	Coconut oil
Palmitic acid	$CH_3 (CH_2)_{14} COOH$	Animal, plant
Stearic acid	$CH_3 (CH_2)_{16} COOH$	Animal, plant
Arachidicacid	$CH_3 (CH_2)_{18} COOH$	Peanut oil

Unsaturated fatty acids

Oleic acid	$CH_3 (CH_2)_7 CH = CH-$ $(CH_2)_7 - COOH$	animal, plant
Linoleic acid	$CH_3(CH_2)_3 (CH_2 CH = CH)_2 (CH2)_7 COOH$	Plant oils
Linolenic acid	$CH_3 (CH_2 - CH = CH)_3$ $(CH_2)_7 COOH$	Linseed oil

Polyunsaturated fatty acids are the precursors for the biosynthesis of prostaglandins.

Physical properties of fatty acids and triglycerides

(i) **Solubility :** They have very low solubility in water. The low molecular weight fatty acids like acetic and butyric acid are miscible with water. High molecular weight fatty acids are soluble in organic solvent like ethers.

(ii) **Formation of Translucent spot on paper :** Place a drop of olive oil upon a piece of ordinary writing paper. Observe the semitransparent appearance of the paper at the point of contact with the fat.

Chemical properties of fatty acids : Unsaturated fatty acids can be halogenated or hydrogenated as follows :

9, 10-Dibromostearic acid

Oleic acid

Stearic·acid

Oleic acid

(Cis-9-Octadecenoic acid)

$$\downarrow \; HNO_2$$

$$\begin{array}{cc} H & (CH_2)_7\text{—COOH} \\ \diagdown \\ C \\ \| \\ C \diagdown \\ (CH_2)_7 \qquad\qquad H \\ | \\ CH_3 \qquad\qquad \text{Elaidic acid} \end{array}$$

(trans-9-octadecenoic acid)

Oxidation of fatty acids

Light, irradiations or metal ion contamination will lead to the production of peroxy radicals in lipids. When this change occurs in a food product, is called oxidative rancidity. Lipid containing food products are protected by the addition of anti-oxidants. Natural antioxidants are vitamin E and ascorbic acid.

Biological membranes : Biological membranes are composed mainly of lipid and protein. Membrane lipids act as permeability barrier, membrane proteins act as pumps, enzymes, receptors and energy transducers.

The major lipids present in biological membrane are phospholipids, glycolipids and cholesterol.

Membrane lipids spontaneously form bimolecular layers.

Circles depict the charged or polar group of lipids

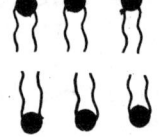

The hydrophobic components face inward.

Basic lipids bilayer model

Acylglycerols

These are esters of glycerol with fatty acids. Palmitic acid stearicacid and oleic acid are common long chain fatty acid present in the human body. The alcoholic hydroxyl groups of glycerol undergo esterification with various fatty acids.

$$CH_2O—\overset{\overset{O}{\|}}{C}—R1$$
$$HC—OH$$
$$CH_2OH$$

$$CH_2O—\overset{\overset{O}{\|}}{C}—R1$$
$$HC—O—\overset{\overset{O}{\|}}{C}—R2$$
$$CH_2OH$$

$$CH_2—O—\overset{\overset{O}{\|}}{C}—R1$$
$$HC—O—\overset{\overset{O}{\|}}{C}—R2$$
$$CH_2 - O - \overset{\overset{O}{\|}}{C} - R3$$

1-acylglycerol   2, 2-Diacylglycerol   Triacylglycerol

Triacylglycerols (Triglycerides) are the principal storage fats in humans.

Triglycerides are hydrolyzed to glycerol and free fatty acids by hormone sensitive lipase enzymes.

Phosphoglycerides

They are phosphate esters of diglycerides

e.g.
$$CH_2 OH$$
$$H\text{-}C — OH$$
$$H_2C — O — \overset{\overset{O}{\|}}{\underset{OH}{P}} — OH \text{ Glycerol -3 - phosphate}$$

when two fatty acids are esterified to glycerol 3 - phosphate, phosphatidic acid is produced.

$$CH_2—O—\overset{\overset{O}{\|}}{C}—R_1$$
$$HC—O—\overset{\overset{O}{\|}}{C}—R_2$$
$$H_2C—O—\overset{\overset{O}{\|}}{\underset{OH}{P}}\text{-}OH$$

Phosphatidic acid

Phosphatidic acid is an intermediate in the synthesis of various other phosphoglycerides.

$$H_2C—O—\overset{\overset{O}{\|}}{C}—R_1$$
$$HC—O—\overset{\overset{O}{\|}}{C}—R_2$$
$$H_2C—O—\overset{\underset{OH}{|}}{P}—O—CH_2—CH_2—\overset{\overset{CH_3}{|}}{\underset{CH_3}{\underset{|}{N}}}—CH_3$$

Choline

Phosphatidylcholine (Lecithin)

It is present in RBCs & lung. It plays an important role in reducing surface tension in lung alveoli. It is an effective surface active agent. Deficiency of lecithin in the lung causes respiratory distress Syndrome (RDS) in premature infants.

$$CH_2—O—CO—R_1$$
$$HC—O—CO—R_2$$
$$CH_2—O—P—Choline$$
Lecithin

Phospholipase A_2
Present in
Cobra Venom

$$CH_2—O—CO—R_1$$
$$HC—OH$$
$$CH_2—O—P—Choline$$
Lysolecithin

Lysolecithin has hemolytic effect.

$$CH_2—O—\overset{\overset{O}{\|}}{C}—R_1$$
$$HC—O—\overset{\overset{O}{\|}}{C}—R_2$$
$$H_2C—O—\overset{\underset{OH}{|}}{P}—O—CH_2—\underset{COOH}{\underset{|}{CH}}—NH_2$$

Ethanolamine

Phosphatidylethanolamine (cephalin)

Cephalin occur in blood platelets and constitute the platelet factor for coagulation.

$$CH_2—O—\overset{\overset{O}{\|}}{C}—R_1$$
$$HC—O—\overset{\overset{O}{\|}}{C}—R_2$$
$$CH_2—O—\overset{\underset{OH}{|}}{P}—O—CH_2—\underset{NH_2}{\underset{|}{CH}}—COOH$$

Serine

Phosphatidylserine

It is present in the brain.

Sphingolipids

Sphingolipids contain sphingosine

Sphingolipids are prsent in nervous system as components of myelin.

Ceramides : Consist of a fatty acid bound to sphingosine.

Cerebrosides : They are Glycolipids having sphingosine, fatty acid combination but a glucose or galactose molecule is attached to ceramide on the place of choline. They are present in the brain.

Gangliosides contain ceramide attached to an oligosaccharide that contains N-acetylneuraminic acid. Sulfatides are sulfated cerebrosides.

Lipoproteins

Lipids must bind to proteins to make them water soluble for transport in the blood. There are many lipoproteins present in our body.

e.g. Chylomicrons
Very-low-density-lipoproteins (VLDL)
Lowdensity lipoproteins (LDL)
High-density lipoproteins (HDL)

Chylomicrons : Consist mainly of trigly-cerides with small amounts of cholesterol, phospholipids and proteins. After a lipid rich meal, the blood appears milky due to the high concentration of chylomicrons. Heparin, stimulates lipoprotein lipase and clears chylomicron from the blood. The inherited absence of lipoprotein lipase causes hyperchylomicronemia (Fredrickson's type I hyperlipoproteinemia).

VLDL are synthesized in the liver and is elevated in type IV hyperlipoproteinemia

LDL is elevated in type II hyperlipoproteinemia HDL level decreases in cardiovascular diseases.

CHEMICAL CONSTANTS FOR FATS

Analytical methods

Saponification number : It is the number of milligram of potassium hydroxide required to saponify 1 gram of fat or oil. An oil with a higher amount of short chain fatty acids gives a higher Saponification number.

Acid number

It is the number of milligram of potassium hydroxide required to neutralize the free fatty acid of one gram of fat. Acid number detects the extent of hydrolysis and liberation of free faty acid that has occured in fats.

Iodine number

It is the amount of Iodine in grams absorbed by 100 gram of fat. The degree of unsaturation of fat is given by the iodine number.

Acetyl number

It is the milligram of potassium hydroxide required to neutralize the acetic acid from 1 gram of the acetylated fat Gas liquid chromatography can be used for the detection and estmation of fatty acids.

DISEASES RELATED TO LIPID METABOLISM

Hyperlipoproteinemias

Their common causes are diabetesmellitus, hypothyroidism and high intake of saturated fat.

With normal cells, LDL in high concentrations saturates the LDL membrane receptors, which signals the cell to stop synthesizing cholesterol. In homozygous hypercholesterolemia there is lack of functional LDL membrane receptors,therefore, even high levels of circulating LDL fail to shut of cholesterol biosynthesis.

Persons with heterozygous hypercholesterolemia have a reduced number of functional LDL receptors.

QUESTIONS

1. Define the term lipids
2. What are the physical and chemical properties of lipids ?
3. How do you classify lipids ?
4. What are the chemical constants for fats ?
5. What are the diseases which occur due to disorders of lipid metabolism ?

5

VITAMINS

Vitamins are organic substances required in small amounts by the body. They do not themselves yield energy they are essential to complete the metabolism energy yielding substances. Deficiency of vitamins produce metabolic disorders. Deficiency of vitamin in the body occurs due to lack of vitamin in the diet or due to disturbances in the absorption of vitamins. Vitamins act as co-enzyme in the metabolic reactions.

Vitamins are classified into two main groups.

(a) Fat soluble vitamins

e.g.   Vitamin A, D, E and K

(b) Water soluble vitamins

e.g.   B1, B2, B3, B6, B12, vit C etc.

Fat soluble vitamins

Vitamin A (Retinoids)

Vitamin A_1 (Retinol)

Vitamin A_2 (3-dehydroretinol)

Sources : β-carotene (in plant), liver, fish and milk.

Functions

Vitamin A is essential for the normal development of epithelial cell through out the body.

Deficiency   also   causes   xerophthalmia   (Dryness   and ulceration of cornea) and night blindness. Vitamin A is essential for the synthesis of light sensitive pigment called rhodopsin. It is required for the biosynthesis of mucopolysaccharide.

Daily requirement : 5000 IU

Excess intake of vitamin A is harmful to the body. Joint pain, loss of hair, thickening of long bones, dry scaly lips etc occurs.

Vitamin D (Solar Vitamin)

Ergocalciferol (Vitamin D_2)

7-dehydrocholesterol

↓ Photolysis

Cholecalciferol

↓ Liver hydroxylase

25 -Hydroxycholecalciferol

↓ Renal 1α-hydroxylase

1, 25 - dihydroxy cholecalciferol

Vitamin D regulates calcium metabolism.

It facilitates the absorption of calcium and phosphate into plasma by small intestine. It promotes the mobilization of Ca++ and PO4 from bone.

It decreases the excretion of Ca++ by the kidney.

Deficiency causes ricketsia inchildren and osteomalacia in adults.

Excess intake of vitamin D causes hypercalcemia and deposition of calcium in soft tissues like lungs, kidney, heart and blood vessels.

Daily requirement : 400 IU/day

Vitamin E (Tocopherols)

Sources : Vegetable oils, grams, leafy vegetable

α-tocopherol is the most active. It is an anti-oxidant. It prevents the formation of toxic oxidation products from unsaturated fatty acids. Polyunsaturated fatty acid are easily attacked by molecular oxygen and forms peroxides. It protects erythrocytes.

Daily requirement : 10-30 mg/day. Deficiency of Vitmain E can cause hemolysis and neurological damage.

Vitamin K

Vitamin K is present in liver, alfalfa leaves and vegetable oils;

    Vitamin K1 (Phytonadione)

    Vitamin K2 (Menaquinone)

    Vitamin K3 (Menadione)

    Vitamin K is essential for the biosynthesis of clotting factors.

    Daily requirement : 0.5 - 1.5 mg/kg

Deficiency symptoms

    Gastric bleeding

    Hematuria

    Hypoprothrombinemia

    Post-operative hemorrhage

    Excess intake of vitamin K acauses

    Chest pain, liver and spleen abnormality.

Water Soluble Vitamins

Thiamine (B1)

Sources : Bran, yeast, egg yolk, liver, meat

Requirement : 1 mg/day

Functions

Thiamine is converted to thiamine pyrophosphate (TPP) in the liver.

    TPP helps in the oxidative decarboxylation of pyruvic acid to acetyl CoA.

    TPP also catalyzes the oxidative decarboxylation of α-ketoglutaric acid to succinyl CoA. Thus it promotes the oxidation of glucose via the Kreb's cycle. It is also required for the hexose-monophosphate shunt pathway.

Deficiency diseases

Vitamin B_1 deficiency causes Beri-beri (Polyneuritis) Thiamine deficiency increases the blood pyruvic acid level and loss of appetite.

Severe deficiency of thiamine causes disorder of carbohydrate metabolism in the heart and blood vessels causing congestive heart failure (wet beriberi).

Riboflavin

Vitamin B2

Sources : Yeast, leafy vegetables, germinating seeds, liver, fish, peas, beans, rice bran.

Requirement : 1.6 - 1.2 mg/day

Function : Riboflavin exists in two forms in the body; they are flavin mononucleotide and flavin adenine dinucleotide (FMN, FAD). They help in the dehydrogenation reaction.

Deficiency symptoms

Corneal vascularisation, cataract, dimness of vision, angular stomatitis, dermatitis, burning feet syndrome and ulceration of lips.

Nicotinamide (Niacin)

Sources : Meat, grains, yeast, fish, cheese, liver

Daily Requirement : 13 mg/day

Function : Nicotinamide is an important constituent of two coenzymes, coenzyme I (NAD) and Coenzyme II (NADP).

Nicotinamide adenine dinucleotide (NAD) and Nicotinamide adenine dinucleotide phosphate (NADP) play an important role in the transport of hydrogen. Thus nicotinamide helps in the oxidation - reduction reactions in the biological system.

Deficiency symptoms

Pellagra (roughskin dermatitis), gastro-intestinaldisturbances, polyneuritis, hallucination, headache and lethargy.

Pyridoxine (Vitamin B6)

Sources : Yeast, liver, egg yolk, peas, soyabean

Requirement : 1-2 mg/day

Function

Pyridoxin is very essential for protein metabolism. In the body it exists in two forms (Pyridoxal phosphate and Pyridoxamine Phosphate) and both form help in the transamination reaction.

Pyridoxine is essential for hemoglobin synthesis. It is required for the synthesis of gamma amino butyric acid (GABA).

Deficiency syndrome

Polyneuritis, stomatitis, convulsion and anemia

Folic acid (Vitamin M, Vitamin B)

Sources : Yeast, green leaves, fruits, liver.

Requirement : 50 ug/day

Functions

Folic acid is very essential for cell division and growth.

Folic acid is converted to tetrahydrofolic acid in the body. Tetrahydrofolic acid is required for the biosynthesis of pyrimidine and purine bases.

It is also required for the formation of red blood cells.

Deficiency Symptoms

Macrocytic anemia, pellagra

Cyanocobalamin (Vitamin B_{12})

Sources : Liver and other non-vegetarian food.

Requirement : 1 ug/day

Function

Cyanocobalamin is required for the biosynthesis of nucleic acids. It acts as co-enzyme. It is essential for the development of epithelial cells. It has lipotropic action. It promotes the conversion of methylmalonyl CoA to succinyl CoA. Formation and function of myelinated nerve fibre requires B_{12}.

Deficiency symtpoms

Pernicious anemia

Peripheral neuritis

Intrinsic factor : Intrinsic factor is a glycoprotein present in gastric secretion. Intrinsic factor is very essential for the intestinal absorption of cyanocobalamine or vitamin B_{12}.

Ascorbic acid (Vitamin C)

Sources : Citrus fruits, tomatoes, potatoes, green vegetables.

Requirement : 25-75 mg/day

Functions

Vitamin C is essential for the conversion of folicacid to folinic acid and therefore, is necessary for the growth and maturation of red blood cells. It regulates the synthesis of the intracellular "cement substances" of the capillaries. Bleeding in scurvy is also explained on the basis of lack of intracellular cementing material. Vitamin C helps in the conversion of ferric salts into ferrous salts.

It is required for the metabolism of amino acids and carbohydrate.

Deficiency symptoms

Scurvy, anemia, reduced glucose tolerance.

Pantothenic acid

Sources : Yeast, liver, eggs, peanut, whole wheat.

Requirement : 5 mg/day

Functions

It acts as an essential constituent of co-enzyme A. It plays an important role in the biosynthesis of acetylcholine, hemoglobin, steroids and lipids.

Deficiency symptoms

Neuromuscular degeneration, adrenocortical insufficiency malaise, nausea, flatulence and vomiting.

Biotin (vitamin H)

Sources : Yeast, peas, cereals, liver and eggs.

Requirements : 100 ug/day

Functions

It helps in the fixation of carbondioxide. It is required for the biosynthesis of fatty acids.

Deficiency symptoms

Exfoliative dermatitis, atropy of the lingual papillae, muscular pain, anorexia and disturbed erythropoiesis.

Inositol

Sources : Fruits, cereals, liver
Requirement : 1 g/day

Functions

It is essential for fat metabolism. It acts as a lipotropic agent. It is a constituent of phosphatidyl inositol and phospholipid of the cell membrane.

Rutin (Vitamin P)

It reduces the capillary permeability. Hence, can be used along with vitamin C.

QUESTIONS

1. Define the term vitamins
2. Classify vitamins based upon their solubility.
3. What are the biochemical role of vitamin A ?
4. What happens to the body when excess Vitamin A is consumed ?
5. Explain the role of vitamin D in calcium metabolism.
6. Write the name of an anti-oxidant fat soluble vitamin.
7. What is meant by Beri-Beri ? How can you prevent the occurence of Beri-Beri ?
8. Which vitamins act as co-enzymes during dehydrogenation reaction ?
9. Which vitamin is very essential for transamination reaction ?
10. Write the name of a vitamin which is very essential for purine and pyrimidine biosynthesis.
11. What are the uses of cyanocobalamin ?
12. What is meant by scurvy ? How do you prevent the symptoms of scurvy ?

6

MINERALS AND WATER
IN LIFE PROCESS

Tissues as well as cardiovascular system of human body contain large amount of water and smaller amounts of inorganic salts. These inorganic salts regulate distribution of water through out the body and also play a vital role in the metabolic reactions in the body. Minerals are concerned with the following functions :

    (a) Osmotic pressure

    (b) Cell permeability

    (c) Water distribution

    (d) Generation of electrical potential

    (e) Co-factors in enzymatic reactions

Minerals balance in the body

It depends upon the following conditions

    (a) Amount of minerals present in food

    (b) Efficiency of absorption from gastrointestinal tract

    (c) Utilization and storage of minerals by tissues

    (d) Removal of minerals from the body through the urine, feces and sweat.

The important minerals present in the body are sodium, potassium, calcium, phosphorus and magnesium. Some elements are required in minute quantity and are called trace elements e.g. iron, iodine, copper, cobalt and zinc,

POTASSIUM

Source : Drinking water, beefliver, bananas, pineapple, Potatoes

Requirements : 4 g/day

Functions

(a) Potassium is an important cation in extracellular fluid

(b) It regulates the acid-base balance and nerve function

(c) It helps in muscular activity.

Low Serum potassium : Occurs in post-operative illness malnutrition, diarrhoea, over activity of adrenal cortex and also during diuretic theapy.

High serum potassium : Concentration is caused by potassium sparing diuretics.

High level of potassium produces cardiac arrest and small bowel ulcers.

SODIUM

Source : Cooked food, salted food, bread, cheese, whole grains, carrots, cauliflower, egg., legumes, milk, radish

Requirements

Normal healthy person 5-15 g/day

Patients of hypertension 1 g/day

Functions

(a) Sodium is the major element of extracellular fluid

(b) It is associated with chloride and bicarbonate in the regulation of acid base balance of the body.

(c) Sodium is essential to maintain the osmotic pressure

(d) It protects the body against excessive fluid loss.

(e) It plays an important role in the permeability of cells.

Excess intake of sodium chloride may produce the following symptoms

(i) Hypertension

(ii) Oedema

    (iii) Lipemia

    (iv) Nephrosis

    (v) Anemia

CALCIUM

Source : Milk

Requirement : 400-800 mg/day; During Pregnancy & lactation additional 500 mg is given/day

    Calcium is the most abundant macromineral present in the body. 90% of calcium is present in the bone and teeth and is deposited as calcium phosphate. This deposited calcium is not a permanent one but it will dissolve and re-deposited. About 700 mg of calcium may enter and leave the bones each day.

Calcium absorption and Vitamin D

Vitamin D is essential for the absorption of calcium from intestine.

Functions of calcium

    1. It is essential for the activity of many enzymes

    2. It is required for the blood coagulation.

    3. It is also essential for muscle contractility and normal neuromuscular activity.

Blood calcium

Parathyroid glands are sensitive to the level of circulating calcium.

    Parathyroid gland maintains the constant blood calcium level

PHOSPHORUS

Source : Milk

Requirement : 1.5 g/day

    Phosphorus is present in every cell. 80%, is present in bones and teeth.

    10% in combination with carbohydrate, protein and lipid. Remaining 10% in other parts of the body.

Functions

    (i) It is important for the formation of energy rich phosphate such as adenosine triphosphate

    (ii) It is also a constituent of many enzymes

    (iii) It is an important constituent of phospholipid

    (iv) HPO_4 and H_2PO_4 are required for the maintainence of acid-base stability of blood.

Hypophosphatemia : Occurs due to excess use of aluminium hydroxide as an antacid.

Uncontrolled metabolic acidosis can lead to excessive phosphate loss in the urine. The symptom of hypophosphatemia is muscle weakness and deformity of bones.

MAGNESIUM

Sources : Soyabean, peas, nuts.

Requirements : 300-350 mg/day

Functions

    1. Magnesium is required for the activation of many enzymes involved in the carbohydrate metabolism.

    2. It is also required for the prevention of calcium oxalate stone formation in the kidney.

Deficiency symptoms : Deficiency symptoms are muscle twitch, convulsion, and cardiac arrhythmia.

In diabetes mellitus and acidosis magnesium loss is more from the body.

Trace elements

These are the elements which are required in minute quantities for the body, e.g., Iron, copper, Iodine, manganese, cobalt, zinc. and molybdenum.

IRON

Sources : Organ meat, liver, egg yolk, fish, wheat, green vegetables.

Requirement : 10-18 mg/day

Functions

1. Iron is essential for cellular respiration.
2. Iron is required for the synthesis of iron containing proteins like hemoglobin, myoglobin and cytochrome.

Absorption of iron

Iron in the food is present in the ferric state. In presence of low gastric pH or vitamin C ferric iron is converted into ferrous state in the stomach. Ferrous form of the iron is absorbed into the mucosal cell. The absorption is controlled by ferritin protein present in the mucosal cell. Iron enters the plasma in ferrous form and combines with a glycoprotein called transferrin.

Transferrin is utilized by various organs like liver, bone-marrow, muscle, & other tissues for synthesizing iron ontaining proteins.

Deficiency Symptoms

(i) Microcytic hypochromic anemia
(ii) Decreased immunocompetence.

Toxic effects of iron

Excess iron in the body leads to haemochromatosis in which iron deposits are found in abnormally high levels in many tissues. This can lead to liver, pancreatic and cardiac dysfunction as well as pigmentation of skin.

COPPER

Requirement : 0.05 - 2.5 mg/day

Functions

(i) Copper functions as a co-factor for many enzymes like cytochrome C oxidase, dopamine β-hydroxylase superoxide dismutase and monoamine oxidase.
(ii) It is required for the bisosynthesis of hemoglobin.

Deficiency Symptoms

(i) Anemia
(ii) Hypercholesterolemia

   (iii) Fragility of large arteries

   (iv) Menke's syndrome

IODINE

Source : Sea-food

Requirement : 100-200 µg/day (100 microgram/day)

Functions

1. Iodine is necessary for the formation of thyroid hormone
2. It is obtained from diet in the form of inorganic iodide (which depends upon the nature of soil)
3. The ingested iodine is rapidly absorbed through the digestive tract and taken up by thyroid gland.
4. In the thyroid gland iodine is converted to organic iodine containing compound namely thyroxine.
5. Thyroid hormones increase the oxygen uptake of all tissues.

DEFICIENCY

Deficiency of iodine affect the development of all tissues. The thyroid gland undergoes compensatory enlargement in order to extract iodine from the blood more efficiently. Thyroid gland accumulates iodine poor colloid with its follicles. This causes swelling of thyroid gland. Cretinism occurs in children due to iodine deficiency. Cretinism is characterized by mental retardation, slow body development and dwarfism. Goiter can be prevented by using iodine salt.

MANGANESE

Sources : Vegetables, fruits, nuts

Daily requirement : 4 mg/day

Functions

Manganese is a cofactor for metalloenzymes such as hydrolases, isocitrate dehydrogenase, kinases, ATPases, peptidase, choline esterase, decarboxylases and transferases.

Deficiency

Manganese deficiency decreases the synthesis of oligosaccharide, glycoproteins, and proteoglycans.

COBALT

Source : Present in cyanocobalamin
Requirement : 1.1 mg/body

Function

As a constituent of vitamin B_{12}

ZINC

Sources : Animal protein (meat, eggs, seafood, milk)
Requirement : 15 mg/day

Function

Zinc is a co-factor for nearly 80 enzymes for e.g. alcohol dehydrogenase, DNA & RNA polymerase etc.

Deficiency

Zinc deficiency causes growth retardation, hypogonadism, alopecia, cirrhosis of liver cells and poor apetite.

MOLYBDENUM

Daily Requirement : 0.15-0.5 mg/day

Function

It acts as a co-factor of metalloenzymes like xanthine oxidase, aldehyde oxidase and sulfite oxidase.

Role of water in life process

Water constitutes 45-60% of the body weight. The average % of water for men is 55%, for women it is 50%. Water is distributed in two compartments.

    (a) Extracellular compartment (Plasma, Interstitial fluid)

(b) Intracellular compartment

Factors which influence distribution of water

Water is retained in the body in constant amount. Osmotic force control the amount of fluid in the various compartments of the body.

The osmotic force is maintained by solutes present in the body. Thus solutes are very essential for water distribution, retention and also for maintaining acid-base balance of body.

For example : Organic compound of smaller molecular size like glucose, aminoacids etc. diffuse freely across cell membrane and thus aid in retaining of water in the body.

Protein substances help in distribution of fluid from one compartment of body to other.

Inorganic electrolytes are very essential for retention and distribution of water in the body.

Hence, electrolytes, glucose etc. are given by intravenous route whenever there is dehydration due to severe vomiting or diarrhoea.

QUESTIONS

1. What are the major functions of minerals in our body ?
2. What are the functions of potassium in our body ? Which group of drugs cause potassium loss from the body ?
3. Which is the major element present in extracellular fluid ?
4. What happens when sodium chloride is consumed in excess quantity along with food materials ?
5. What are the functions of calcium ? How parathyroid hormone controls the level of blood calcium ?
6. Write the major functions of phosphorous in our body.
7. What are trace elements ?
8. What do you understand by the term microcytic anemia ?
9. Explain the absorption, distribution and storage of iron in the body.

10. Write the biochemical role of copper in the body.
11. What is meant by cretinism ? How can you prevent the occurence of cretinism ?

7

ENZYMES

Enzymes are protein in nature. Their main function is catalysis of chemical reactions in living systems. Some enzymes may contain, in addition to protein, other non-protein organic groupings or metallic ions. The protein part of enzymes is called the apoenzyme. The non-protein part is called as co-enzyme. Most of the co-enzyme contain the water soluble B-complex group of vitamins as component parts of their structure. The metal ion associated with an enzyme is called a Co-factor.

Some enzymes exist in more than one structural form in the same biological system/species, such enzymes are called as isoenzymes.

Proenzyme : Many proteins are manufactured and secreted from their cells of origin in the form of inactive precursor protein known as Proproteins. When the proproteins are enzymes the proteins are known as proenzymes or zymogens.

e.g.   Proinsulin
        Pepsinogen

ENZYME NOMENCLATURE

The name of an enzyme consists of two parts : first, the name of the substrate; the second portion of the name describes the type of reaction. International Union of Biochemists (IUB) has assigned a recommended name for each enzyme.

e.g.   Alcohol dehydrogenase

        here Alcohol is the substrate name, dehydrogenase describes the type of reaction.

Each enzyme has a systemic code number (E.C.)

This code number indicate the class (first digit), subclass (second digit), and subsubclass (third digit). The fourth digit indicate the specificity of the enzyme. For exxample E.C. 2.7.1.1 indicates.

Class 2   (A transferase)

Subclass 7   (Transfer of phosphate)

Sub-subclass 1   (An alcohol function as the PO_4 acceptor)

Final digit 1   (Enzyme hexokinase)

Enzymes are classified into six major types depending upon the types of reaction catalysed by them.

I. OXIDOREDUCTASES

This group of enzyme include dehydrogenases, oxidases and peroxidases.

They catalyse oxidoreducto reactions between two substrates, S and S'.

$$\text{S-Reduced + S'-oxidised} \xrightarrow{E} \text{S-oxidised+S'reduced}$$

e.g. (i) $\text{Alcohol+NAD} \xrightarrow{\text{Alcohol dehydrogenase}} \text{Aldehyde + NADH + H}$

(ii) $\text{4 Reduced cytochrome } C+O_2+2H_2 \xrightarrow{\text{Cytochrome Oxidase}} \text{4 Oxidised cytochrome } + 2H_2O$

(iii) $\text{2 mole } H_2O_2 \xrightarrow{\text{Catalase}} O_2 + 2H_2O$

II. TRANSFERASES

These enzymes catalyze the transfer of a group (G) other than hydrogen between a pair of substrates, S and S'

$$\text{S - G + S'} \xrightarrow{E} \text{S + S' - G}$$

e.g. Kinases which transfer phosphate from ATP to other compound.

These enzymes catalyze the transfer of one carbon group, aldehyde, ketone, acyl, alkyl and sulphur group.

Enzymes catalyzing the transfer of phosphate containing groups e.g. Hexokinase.

$$\text{ATP + D-hexose} \xrightarrow{\text{Hexokinase}} \text{ADP + D-hexose 6 phosphate}$$

$$\text{Acetyl CoA + Choline} \xrightarrow[\text{Acyltransferase}]{\text{Choline}} \text{Acetylcholine + CoA}$$

III. HYDROLASES

These enzymes catalyze the hydrolysis of compounds. Proteolytic enzymes, lipases and amylase belongs to this group.

e.g. $\text{Acetyl choline + H}_2\text{O} \xrightarrow{\text{Cholinesterase}} \text{Choline + Acetic acid}$

IV. LYASES

These enzymes catalyze the non-hydrolytic removal of group from substrates.

e.g. (i) Fructose 1, 6 $\xrightarrow{\text{Aldolase}}$ D-Glyceraldehyde 3-phosphate
       diphosphate   + Dihydroxyacetone phosphate

(ii) L-Malate $\xrightarrow{\text{Fumarase}}$ Fumarate + H$_2$O

V. ISOMERASES

This class of enzyme catalyze cis-trans isomerization, epimerization and racemization.

(i) Trans-retinene $\xrightarrow[\text{isomerase}]{\text{Retinene}}$ cis-retinene

(ii) Galactose $\xrightarrow{\text{Epimerase}}$ Glucose

(iii) L Alanine $\xrightarrow{\text{Alanine Racemase}}$ D-Alanine

(iv) Glyceraldehyde $\xrightarrow[\text{Triosphosphate isomerase}]{}$ Dihydroxy acetone
     3-phosphate   phosphate

VI.   LIGASES (Ligare = to bind)

Ligases catalyze the coupling together of two molecules with the breaking of a pyrophosphate bond in ATP or similar compound. e.g.

$$GTP + Succinate + CoA \xrightarrow[\text{Thiokinase}]{\text{Succinic}} GDP + Succinyl\,COA + P_1$$

| Guanosine | Guanosine |
| Triphosphate | diphosphate |

ISOLATION OF ENZYMES

Purified enzymes are used to study the metabolic pathways. Isolated enzymes are useful to measure the kinetics of a reaction. The chemical structure, and the active site of an enzyme can be studied when the enzyme is in pure form.

The enzyme protein can be extracted from crude protein by precipitation techniques. Electrophoretic techniques are also used to isolate enzymes. Other methods used to isolate enzymes are affinity chromatography, gel filtration and differential centrifugation.

Basic Concept of Enzyme Action

Enzymes are very specific in catalysing particular reaction. Thus they control the metabolic process and normal function of the cell. Each enzyme molecule has an "Active Center" of precisely defined Chemical structure and that the combination with the substrate occurs at this center.

Enzymes are stereospecific in catalyzing a particular reaction. For example lactate dehydrogenase acts on L-lactic acid, the D-isomer is unaffected. Similarly fumarase acts only on the trans fumaric acid and has no effect on the cis-fumaric acid.Maltase catalyzes the hydrolysis of α-glucoside but not β-glucoside.

Active site (Catalytic site, substrate site)

Enzymes contain functional groups like SH, OH and NH_2 groups which are necessary for catalytic action. If any chemical reagents react with these functional groups then the enzymatic activity is frequently lost. e.g. p. chloromercuribenzoate reacts with -SH group of urease and causes complete inactivation. The above information indicate that these groups are important points of attachments for substrate. These specific region of enzyme function as an "active site" (catalytic site, substrate site).

First this type of enzyme substrate complex formation was proposed by Fischer.

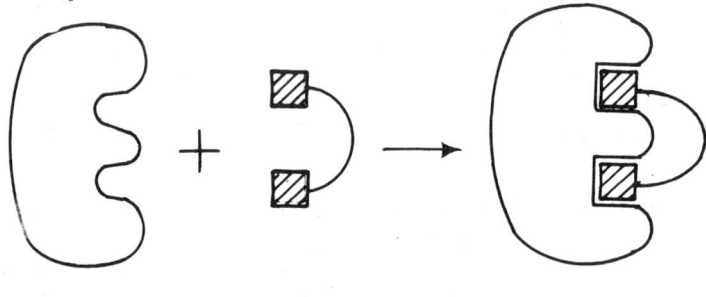

Enzyme   Substrate   Enzyme Substrate complex.

He suggested that it resembles key fitting into a lock. Later Koshland proposed the flexible active site of enzymes. When an enzyme combines with a substrate, conformatiional changes of enzyme occurs. The flexible site theory by Khosland helps to explain how compounds, unrelated to normal substrate for an enzyme can stimulate or inhibit the activity. In the absence of substrate catalytic group and binding group are for away from one another. Approach of substrate induces conformational change and make the groups suitable for binding and catalysis. Substrate analogue does not produce correct conformational change.

Measurement of enzyme activity

The activity of an enzyme may be measured by following the chemical change catalyzed by the enzyme. The enzyme is incubated under proper condition with substrate. Samples are withdrawn at short interval and analysed for the disappearance of substrate or appearance of products.

e.g.   Action of invertase on sucrose can be measured by estimating the appearance of glucose.

Enzyme units : Enzyme units are expressed in micromoles or nanomoles or picomoles of substrate reacting or product formed per minute or per hour under specified assay condition.

Absorption maximum before and after the enzymatic reaction

can be observed at a particular wavelength to measure the enzyme activity.

Factors affecting rate of enzyme action

Many factors influence the rate of enzyme action they are

(i) Substrate concentration

(ii) Enzyme concentration

(iii) Temperature

(iv) pH

(v) Presence of activators

(vi) Presence of inhibitors

Substrate concentration

When the enzyme concentration is kept at a constant value an increase in substrate concentration increases the initial velocity and reaches the maximum value. The velocity increases as the substrate concentration is increased until enzyme is saturated with substrate. The effect of subsrate concentration on the velocity of enzyme catalysed reaction can be represented graphically.

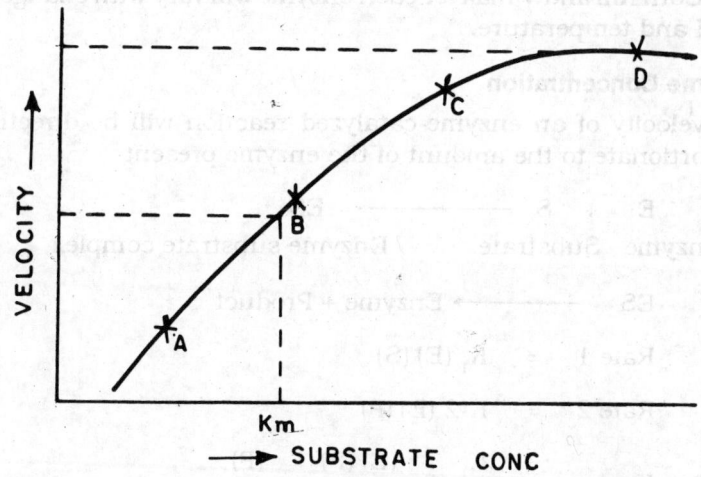

The reaction rate progress slowly then soon it decreases at point beyond D. This indicate that at points A, B and C all the enzyme molecules are not combined with substrate. Therefore, at these points either a decrease or an increase in substrate concentration can alter the rate of reaction. However, point D indicates that all the enzyme molecules are combined with substrate and a further increase in substrate concentration will not cause an increase in the rate of reaction.

The substrate concentration that produces half maximal velocity is termed the Km value or Michaelis constant. It is determined experimentally by plotting velocity versus substrate concentration. When substrate concentration is below Km value, the velocity V depends upon substrate concentration (S). Similarly when the substrate concentration exceeds, Km value, the measured velocity V is maximal V.

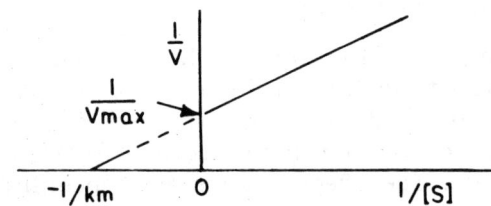

Double-reciprocal or Lineweaver-Burk plot of 1/v versus 1/{s} used for graphic evaluation of Km and V

Both Km and V max for each enzyme will vary with changes in pH and temperature.

Enzyme Concentration

The velocity of an enzyme-catalyzed reaction will be directly proportionate to the amount of the enzyme present.

$$\text{E} \;+\; \text{S} \longrightarrow \text{ES}$$

Enzyme   Substrate   Enzyme substrate complex

$$\text{ES} \longrightarrow \text{Enzyme + Product}$$

$$\text{Rate 1} \;=\; K_1\,(E)\,(S)$$

$$\text{Rate 2} \;=\; K\text{-2}\,(E)\,(P)$$

$$K\,eq \;=\; \frac{K_1}{K_2} \;=\; \frac{(E)\,(P)}{(E)\,(S)} \;=\; \frac{(P)}{(S)}$$

The enzyme concentration thus has no effect on the equilibrium constant.

Temperature

Temperature plays an important role, in the velocity of enzyme catalysed reaction. Over a certain range of temperature, the velocity of enzyme catalyzed reactions increases as temperature rises. The correct ratio by which the velocity changes for a 10°C temperature rise is the Q_{10}, or temperature co-efficient.

The effect of temperature on velocity of enzyme catalyzed reaction can be represented graphically.

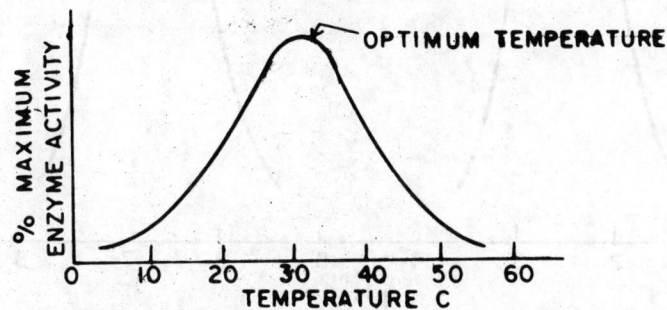

The graph shows that the % activity slowly increases with rise in temperature, however, after certain range, activity decreases due to denaturation of protein.

PH

Slight pH changes affect the ionic state of the enzyme and often that of the substrate also. By measuring the enzyme activity at several pH values, the optimum pH can be determined.

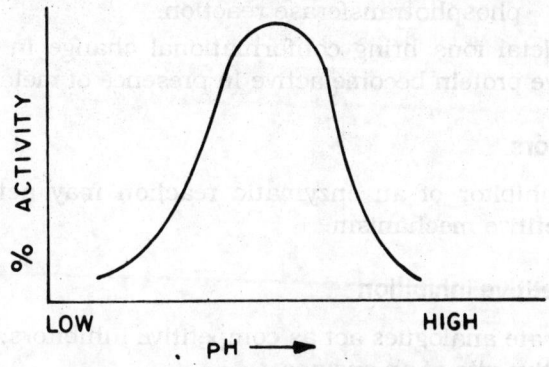

Effect of pH on enzyme activity

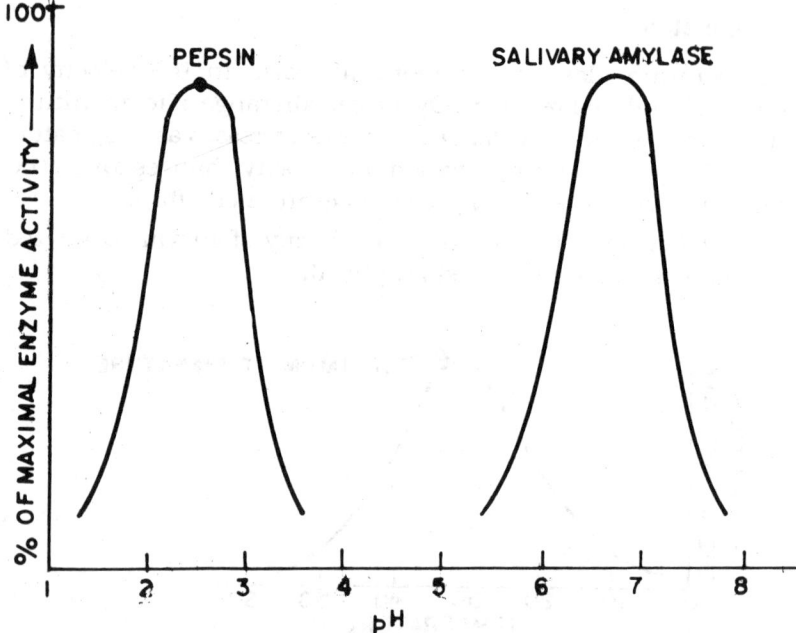

Activators

Many metal ions modify the enzyme catalyzed reaction. Metal ion may undergo valency change during an oxidation-reduction reaction and catalyze the reaction e.g. Fe in cytochrome or catalase undergoes valency change during drug-oxidation.

Metal ions may combine with substrate and metalion substrate complex will act as true substrate

e.g. $Mg++ + ATP \longrightarrow Mg++$ ATP is the true substrate for phosphotransferase reaction.

Metal ions bring conformational change in protein. An inactive protein become active in presence of metal ion.

Inhibitors

The inhibitor of an enzymatic reaction may act by a non-competitive mechanism.

Competitive inhibition

Substrate analogues act as competitive inhibitors. It occurs at the active site of an enzyme.

e.g. 1. Sulfanilamide, a structural analog of p-amino-benzoate
will inhibit folic acid synthesis.

Sulfanilamide inhibits dihydropteroate synthase,
an enzyme responsible for the incorporation of PABA
into dihydropteroic acid, the immediate precursor of
folicacid.

2. Malonic acid is a competitive inhibitor of succinic
dehydrogenase enzyme.

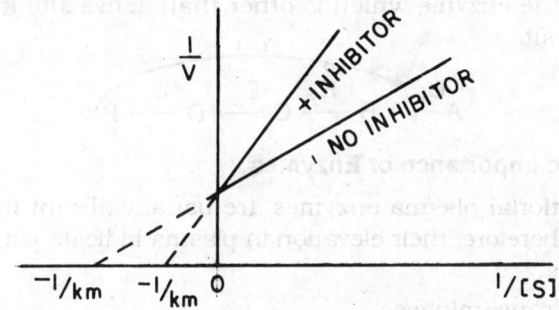

Fig. 7.7 Lineweaver-Burk plot of classic competitive inhibition

Non-competitive inhibition

The inhibitor may not be a substrate analogue and it binds at a
different site. Non-competitive inhibitor lowers the maximal
velocity.

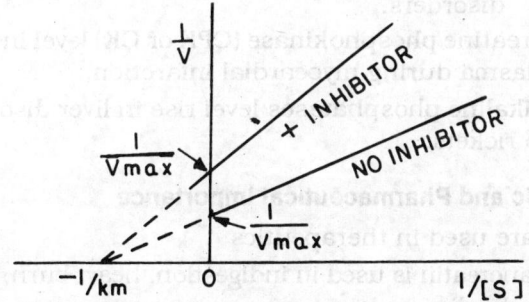

Fig. 7.8 Lineweaver-Burk plot for reversible non-competitive inhibition

Irreversible non-competitive inhibition

Many enzyme "poisons" like iodoacetamide, heavymetal ions
(Ag++, Hg++) Oxidizing agents etc decreases enzyme activity.

The intestinal parasite Ascaris contain pepsin and trypsin inhibitors. Thus the parasitic worm escapes digestion in the intestine.

Allosteric inhibition

It has been observed that product (P) of a series of biochemical reaction. inhibits the enzyme (E_1)required in the first step even though structure (P) is different from A. This type of inhibition is called allosteric inhibition. This is due to the binding of (P) at a site on the enzyme which is other than active site known as allosteric site

$$A \xrightarrow{E_1} B \xrightarrow{E_2} C \xrightarrow{E_3} D \xrightarrow{E_4} P$$

Diagnostic importance of Enzymes

Non-functional plasma enzymes are usually absent in normal plasma. Therefore, their elevation in plasma indicate pathological conditions.

e.g. (a) Transaminases

  (i) SGOT (Serum Glutamate,oxaloacetic Transaminase) or AST (Aspartate aminotransferase) level rises in cardiovascular disease like myocardial infarction.

  (ii) SGPT (Serum Glutamic pyruvic transaminase)

   or

   ALT (Alanine aminotransferase) level rises in liver disorders.

(b) Creatine phosphokinase (CPK or CK) level increases in plasma during myocardial infarction.

(c) Alkaline phosphatases level rise in liver disorders and in rickets.

Therapeutic and Pharmaceutical importance

Enzymes are used in therapeutics

e.g. (a) Pancreatin is used in indigestion, heart burn, flatulence and colic.

(b) Proteases and amylase are useful in dyspepsia.

(c) Streptokinases and urokinase are used in heart attack to dissolve the clot and are given intravenously.

(d) Lipase enzyme is used in pancreatic deficiency state

(e) Aspariginase is used in the treatment of cancer.

QUESTIONS

1. Define the following terms
   (i) Enzymes
   (ii) Pro-enzymes
2. How do you classify enzymes ? Give suitable example for each type.
3. What is active site ?
4. How do you measure the enzyme activity ?
5. What are the various factors which affect the enzyme catalyzed reaction ?
7. Write briefly the competitive and non-competitive inhibition of enzyme activity.
8. What is meant by allosteric inhibition ?
9. What are the significances of enzyme estimation ?
10. What are the therapeutic and pharmaceutical uses of enzymes ?

8

METABOLISM OF PROTEINS

Protein consumption is an index of a country's economic status, because quality protein is the most expensive food. Protein malnutrition leads to poor health, disease and even death.

Proteins are very essential as building blocks of cells. Proteins are required to make enzymes which play a vital role in various other metabolism. Ingested proteins are degraded in the GI tract to smaller units called aminoacids.

Digestion of protein

Digestion of protein begins in the stomach. Hydrolysis of protein is initiated in the stomach by the enzyme pepsin and protease. Pepsin and protease are secreted by cells lining the walls of the stomach, Gastric mucosa secretes hydrochloric acid and mucus also.

The hydrochloric acid is responsible for low pH of gastric juice (pH 1-2). This acidic pH helps in the activity of pepsin in two ways.

1. Pepsin is first secreted as pepsinogen. This pepsinogen is converted to pepsin by pepsin itself at acidic pH. Pepsin preferentially attacks peptide bonds involving residues of aromatic amino acid.

2. Maximum pepsin activity occurs at pH 1-2. Pepsin helps in breaking of large protein molecule to smaller polypeptide chain.

Protein digestion in the small intestine is catalyzed by enzymes secreted by pancreas. Carboxypeptidase, chymotrypsin and trypsin convert polypeptides into small polypeptides and dipeptides. In the small intestine brush border area, smaller polypeptides and dipeptides are converted to free amino acids by peptidases.

Amino acids produced from the protein are absorbed in the form of amino acid through the small intestine and enter into the portal vein and reaches the liver. From the liver aminoacids are supplied to other parts.

Protein utilization

Absorbed aminoacids will be utilized for the biosynthesis of new protein according to the need of the individual cell. A portion of amino acid absorbed is concentrated by liver cell and the remaining portion pass into systemic circulation for other tissues. Amino acids which are in excess of hepatic needs are deaminated and the amino group is utilized for urea formation, and the ketoacids are oxidised to CO_2 and water. Vital proteins like plasma albumin, α, β globulin and fibrinogen are synthesized in the liver.

Mechanisms of protein turnover

(a) When cells die, their components are catabolised and new cells with new components arise in place of dead cells.
(b) Individual protein molecules are degraded and replaced by synthesis without cell death.
(c) It is possible that individual aminoacid is exchanged in intact protein molecules.

Essential aminoacids (indispensable amino acids)

Essential amino acids are not produced in the body. Hence, these amino acids containing protein must be supplied along with other diets. Examples for essential amino acids are

Arginine

Histidine

Isoleucine

Leucine

Lysine

Methionine

Phenylalanine

Threonine

Tryptophan

Valine

The essential amino acids are best provided by proteins of animal origin (e.g. meat, cheese, eggs fish) because plant proteins are deficient in essential amino acids.

Aminoacid Catabolism (Nitrogen catabolism of amino acids)

Amino acids in surplus of needs for protein biosynthesis cannot be stored, nor are they eliminated as such. Amino groups of excess amino acids are removed by oxidative deamination or transamination. The carbon skeletons of amino acids are converted into intermediates which take part in either anabolism or catabolism. Living organisms excrete the amino group in various forms e.g.

Ammonotelic : organisms which excrete free ammonia as the end product of amino group catabolism. (e.g. Fishes).

Uricotelic : Birds and amphibians excrete the end product of nitrogen catabolism as Uric acid.

Ureotelic : Mammals excrete the amino group of amino acids as urea.

Oxidative deamination

An α-amino acid is converted to an α-ketoacid with elimination of aminogroup as ammonia

e.g. :

$$CH_3-\underset{\underset{NH_2}{|}}{\overset{\overset{H}{|}}{C}}-COOH \xrightarrow[\text{Oxidase}]{\text{Aminoacid}} CH_3-\underset{\underset{O}{\|}}{C}-COOH + NH_3$$

Alanine   Pyruvic acid

Transamination

Transamination reaction is catalysed by transaminases or aminotransferases. In the transamination reaction α-amino acid is converted to an α-ketoacid with simultaneous conversion of an α-ketoacid to an α-amino acid occurs.

$$R—CH—NH_2$$
COOH
α-amino acid

Transaminase

Pyridoxine

$$R - C = O$$
COOH

$$R^1$$
$$C = O$$
COOH
α-ketoacid

$$R^1$$
CH - NH$_2$
COOH

Transaminases (SGOT and SGPT) rises in the plasma whenever there is liver and cardiac disease.

Transport of ammonia

In metabolic acidosis ammonia is excreted as ammonium salt

It is excreted as Urea

The ammonia absorbed from the intestine enters into the portal circulation and then to liver cells where it is converted into urea. Because minute amount of ammonia is toxic to the contral nervous system. Toxic symptoms are tremor, blurring of vision, slurring of speech etc.

Urea cycle : The reaction occurs both in mitochondria and cytosol.

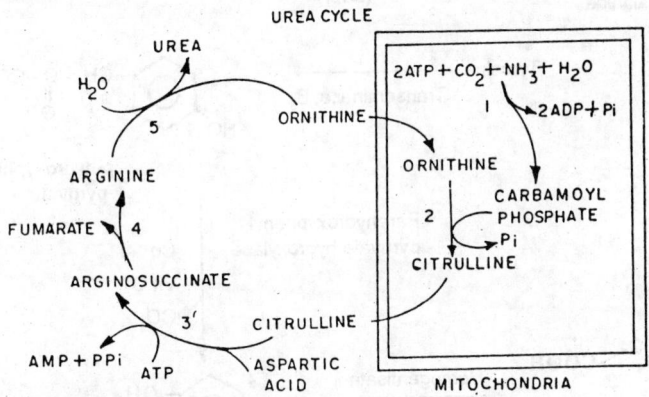

UREA CYCLE

1. Carbamolyphosphate synthetase
2. Ornithine transcarbamoylase
3. Argino succinate synthatase
4. Arginosuccinase
5. Arginase

Disorders of Urea cycle leads to the accumulation of ammonia, vomiting in infancy, avoidance of high protein diet, lethargy and mental retardation.

Glucogenic amino acids (Antiketogenic or Glycogenic)

L-Alanine, L-Arginine, L-Aspartate, L-cystine, L-Glutamate, L-Glycine, L-Histidine, L-Hydroxyproline, L-Methionine, L-proline, L-Serine, L-Threonine and L-valine.

Ketogenic amino acid

L-Leucine

on deamination it gives ketoacid which is utilized for fat synthesis.

Glycogenic and ketogenic aminoacids

L-Isoleucine, L-Lysine, L-Phenylalanine, L-Tryptophan

Metabolism of important aminoacids

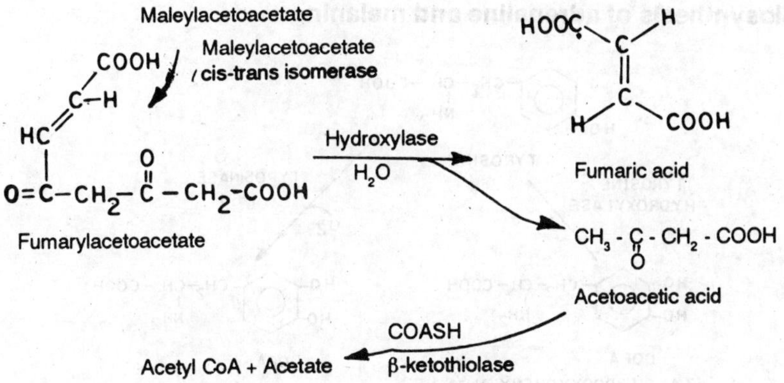

Maleylacetoacetate

COOH
C—H
HC
O
O=C—CH₂— C — CH₂—COOH

Fumarylacetoacetate

Maleylacetoacetate
/ cis-trans isomerase

Hydroxylase
H_2O

HOOC   H
C
C
H   COOH

Fumaric acid

$CH_3 - C - CH_2 - COOH$
           O

Acetoacetic acid

Acetyl CoA + Acetate ← COASH β-ketothiolase

PHENYLKETONURIA

It is an inherited disorder of phenylalanine metabolism. It occurs due to the absence of phenylalanine hydroxylase. In absence of phenylalanine hydroxylase, phenylalanine is converted into phenyl pyruvic acid and phenylacetic acid. Phenylacetic acid is produced due to the oxidative decarboxylation of pyruvic acid Phenylacetate conjugate with glutamine in liver and excreted as phenylglutamine in urine.

Major symptom of phenyl ketonuria is mental retardation

Treatment of Phenylketonuria : Phenylalanine free diet is given.

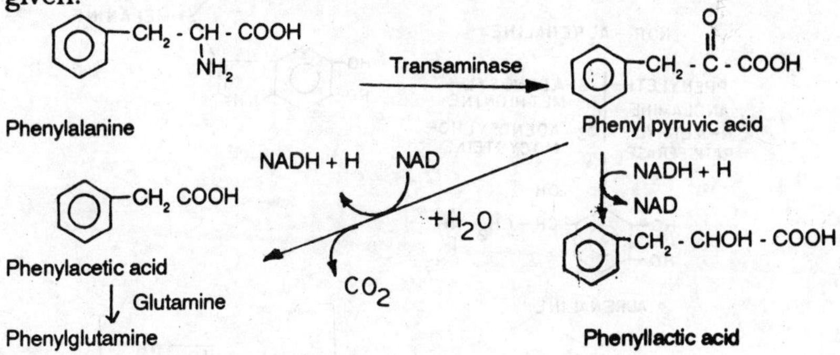

CH₂ - CH - COOH
        NH₂

Phenylalanine

Transaminase →

O
CH₂ - C - COOH

Phenyl pyruvic acid

CH₂ COOH

Phenylacetic acid

↓ Glutamine

Phenylglutamine

NADH + H   NAD

$+H_2O$

CO_2

NADH + H
NAD

CH₂ - CHOH - COOH

Phenyllactic acid

Biosynthesis of adrenaline and melanin

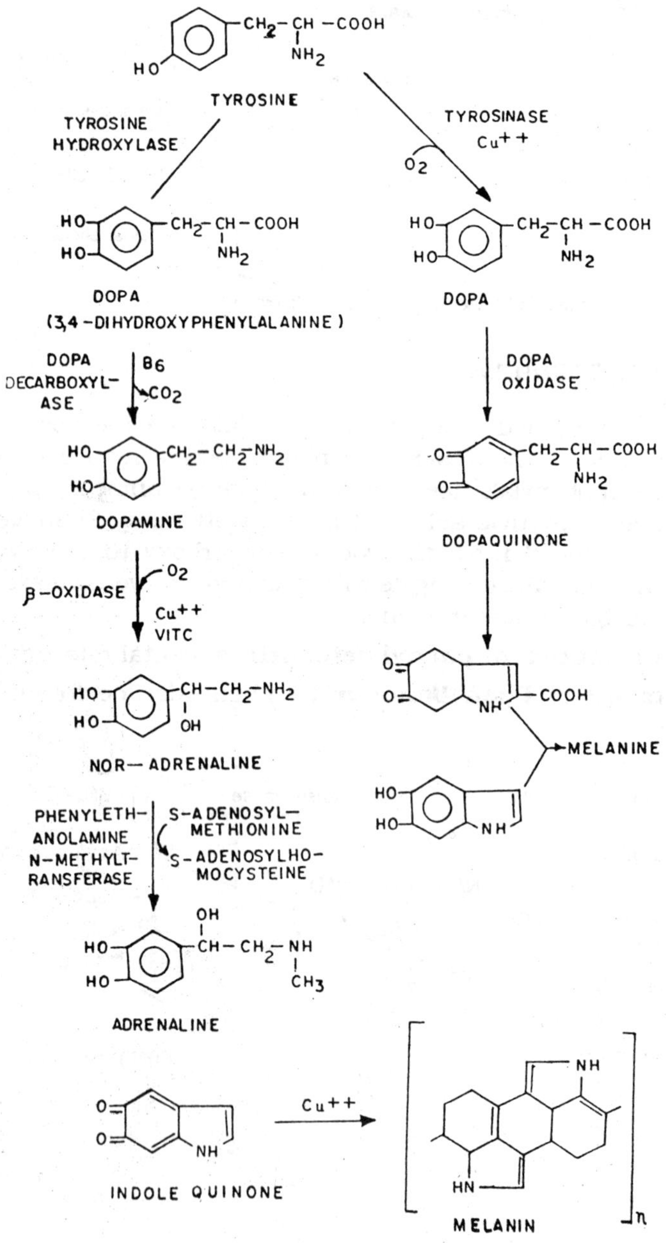

TYROSINE

TYROSINE HYDROXYLASE

TYROSINASE
Cu^{++}
O_2

DOPA
(3,4 –DIHYDROXYPHENYLALANINE)

DOPA

DOPA DECARBOXYL– ASE B_6 CO_2

DOPA OXIDASE

DOPAMINE

DOPAQUINONE

β –OXIDASE O_2 Cu^{++} VITC

NOR– ADRENALINE

PHENYLETH– ANOLAMINE N–METHYLT– RANSFERASE

S–ADENOSYL– METHIONINE
S–ADENOSYLHO– MOCYSTEINE

MELANINE

ADRENALINE

INDOLE QUINONE Cu^{++}

MELANIN

Tyrosine is also utilised for the production of thyroid hormones triiodothyronine and thyroxine.

Nor. adrenaline acts as a neurotransmitter. Adrenaline and nor-adrenaline are present in adrenalmedulla.

Metabolism of tryptophan

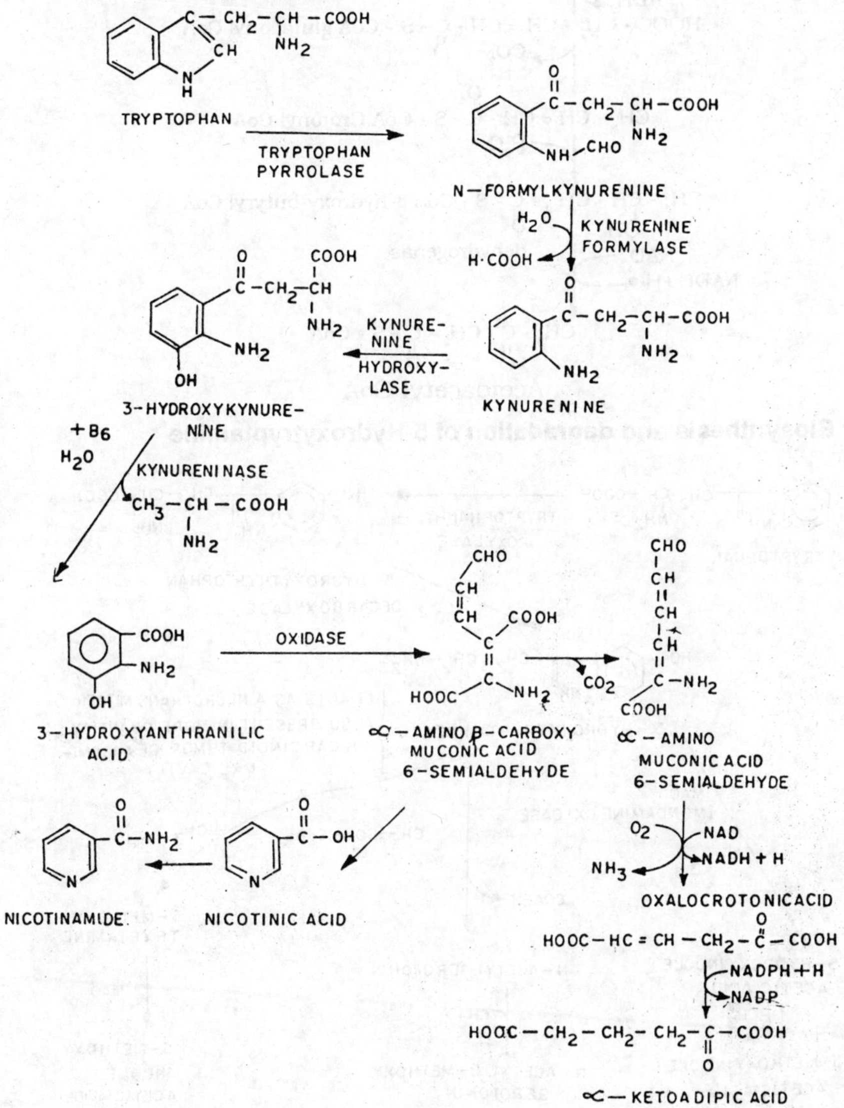

TRYPTOPHAN

TRYPTOPHAN PYRROLASE

N—FORMYLKYNURENINE

H_2O | KYNURENINE FORMYLASE

H·COOH

KYNURENINE

KYNURE-NINE HYDROXY-LASE

3-HYDROXYKYNURE-NINE

+B6 H_2O

KYNURENINASE

$CH_3-CH-COOH$ | NH_2

3-HYDROXYANTHRANILIC ACID

OXIDASE

α—AMINO β—CARBOXY MUCONIC ACID 6—SEMIALDEHYDE

CO_2

α—AMINO MUCONIC ACID 6—SEMIALDEHYDE

NICOTINAMIDE

NICOTINIC ACID

O_2 | NAD
NADH + H

NH_3

OXALOCROTONICACID

$HOOC-HC=CH-CH_2-\overset{O}{\overset{\shortparallel}{C}}-COOH$

NADPH+H
NADP

$HOOC-CH_2-CH_2-CH_2-\overset{}{\underset{O}{\overset{\shortparallel}{C}}}-COOH$

α—KETOADIPIC ACID

$$HOOC - (CH_2)_3 - \overset{\overset{O}{\|}}{C} - COOH \; \alpha \; ketoadipic \; acid$$

CoA, NAD $\longleftarrow$ | $\quad \alpha$-ketoacid dehydrogenase

NADH + CO_2 $\longleftarrow$

$$HOOC - (CH_2)_3 - \overset{\overset{O}{\|}}{C} - S - CoA \; glutaryl \; CoA$$

FAD $\longrightarrow$ | dehydrogenase

FADH$_2$ $\longleftarrow$

$$HOOC - CH_2 - CH = CH - \overset{\overset{O}{\|}}{C} - S - CoA \; glutaconyl \; CoA$$

$\longrightarrow CO_2$

$$CH_3 - CH = CH - \overset{\overset{O}{\|}}{C} - S - CoA \; Crotonyl \; CoA$$

$\longmapsto H_2O$

$$CH_3 - \underset{\underset{OH}{|}}{CH} - CH_2 - \overset{\overset{O}{\|}}{C} - S - CoA \; \beta\text{-hydroxy-butyryl CoA}$$

NAD $\longrightarrow$ | dehydrogenase

NADH + H $\longleftarrow$

$$CH_3 - \overset{\overset{O}{\|}}{C} - CH_2 - \overset{\overset{O}{\|}}{C} - S - CoA.$$

Acetoacetyl CoA

Biosynthesis and degradation of 5-Hydroxytryptamine

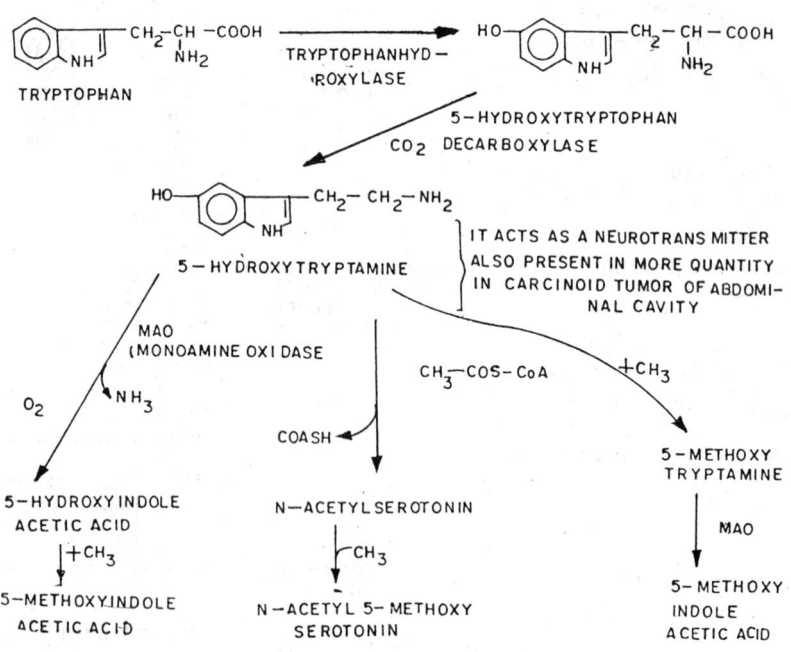

BRANCHED-CHAIN AMiNOACID CATABOLISM

Isoleucine, leucine, and valine are essential amino acids. They are branched chain aminoacids. They are degraded by transamination to α-ketoacids, which are oxidized and decarboxylated to acyl-CoA. The α-ketoacids accumulate and spill into the urine due to the inherited absence of α-ketoacid decarboxylase. Their sweet smell conferred the name of "maple syrup urine disease" to this kind of ketoaciduria. Valine catabolism produces succinyl CoA. Isoleucine catabolism produces propionyl CoA and acetyl CoA.

Basic amino acid metabolism

There are three basic amino acids namely arginine, histidine and lysine.

$$CH = C—CH_2—CH—COOH \qquad CH = C—CH_2—CH_2—NH_2$$

$$\underset{\displaystyle \overset{|}{CH}}{\overset{|}{HN} \quad \overset{\diagdown}{N}} \qquad \overset{|}{NH_2} \quad \xrightarrow{\quad CO_2 \quad} \quad \underset{\displaystyle \overset{|}{CH}}{\overset{|}{HN} \quad \overset{\diagdown}{N}}$$

Histidine   Decarboxylase   Histamine

Histidine on decarboxylation gives histamine. Histamine is an autocoid involved in the allergic and inflammatory reactions in our body.

Methionine and cysteine metabolism

Methionine is an essential aminoacid. It is the precursor of cysteine.

S-adenosylmethionine is formed during metabolism of methionine. S-Adenosylmethionine is an important methyldonor for many biochemical reactions such as methylation of phosphatidylethanolamine to phosphatidylcholine or methylation of nor-adrenaline to adrenaline.

Homocystinuria occurs due to the absence of cystathionine synthase.

Cystathionuria results from the deficiency of cyst-a-thionas.e Both disorders require dietary methionine restriction and cysteine supplementation.

Heterozygous homocystinuria is a common cause of atherosclerosis.

$$CH_3 - S - CH_2 - CH_2 - \overset{\overset{\displaystyle NH_2}{|}}{CH} - COOH \text{ Methionine}$$

ATP
PP$_1$ + P$_1$

$$CH_3 - \underset{\underset{\displaystyle CH_2}{|}}{S} - CH_2 - CH_2 - \overset{\overset{\displaystyle NH_2}{|}}{CH} - COOH$$

Adenine   S-adenosylmethionine

R
R - CH$_3$

$$\underset{\underset{\displaystyle CH_2}{|}}{S} - CH_2 - CH_2 - \overset{\overset{\displaystyle |}{\underset{\displaystyle NH_2}{|}}}{CH} - COOH \text{ S-adenosylhomocysteine}$$

Adenine

H$_2$O
adenosine

$$HS{-}CH_2{-}\overset{\overset{\displaystyle |}{|}}{CH_2}{-}\overset{\overset{\displaystyle |}{\underset{\displaystyle NH_2}{|}}}{CH}{-}COOH \text{ Homocysteine}$$

$$HOOC{-}\overset{\overset{\displaystyle NH_2}{|}}{HC}{-}\overset{\overset{\displaystyle OH}{|}}{CH_2}$$

Cystathionine

H$_2$O   Synthase

$$HOOC{-}\underset{\underset{\displaystyle H_2N}{|}}{HC}{-}CH_2{-}S{-}CH_2{-}CH_2{-}\overset{\overset{\displaystyle |}{\underset{\displaystyle NH_2}{|}}}{CH}{-}COOH \text{ Cystathionine}$$

H$_2$O

Cystathionase

$$HOOC{-}\overset{\overset{\displaystyle NH_2}{|}}{CH}{-}CH_2{-}SH \qquad CH_3{-}CH_2{-}\overset{\overset{\displaystyle O}{\|}}{C}{-}COOH{+}NH_3$$

Cysteine   α-ketobutyrate

Metabolism of glutamic acid, glutamine and proline

Glutamate, glutamine, and proline are all degraded to α-ketoglutarate, a Kreb's cycle intermediate; hence they are glucogenic

$$\begin{array}{l}COOH \\ | \\ CH_2 \\ | \\ CH_2 \\ | \\ HC{-}NH_2 + NH_3 + ATP \longrightarrow \\ | \\ COOH \text{ Glutamic acid}\end{array} \qquad \begin{array}{l}CONH_2 \\ | \\ CH_2 \\ | \\ CH_2 + ADP + Pi + H_2O \\ | \\ CH{-}NH_2 \\ | \\ COOH \text{ Glutamine}\end{array}$$

$$\underset{\text{Glutamic acid}}{HOOC-CH_2-CH_2-\overset{\overset{\displaystyle NH_2}{|}}{CH}-COOH}$$

NADH + ATP

NAD + ADP + Pi

$$H-\underset{\underset{\displaystyle O}{\|}}{C}-CH_2-CH_2-\underset{\underset{\displaystyle NH_2}{|}}{CH}-COOH$$

Glutamate semialdehyde.

H_2O

NADPH

NADP

$$\underset{\text{Proline}}{\underset{\displaystyle NH}{\overset{\displaystyle H_2C-CH_2}{\underset{\displaystyle H_2C\quad CH}{|\quad\ \ |}}-COOH}}$$

$O_2 + \alpha\ KA + CoA$

$Co_2 + Succinyl\ CoA$ Prolylhydroxylase

$$\underset{\text{4-hydroxyproline}}{\underset{\displaystyle NH}{\overset{\displaystyle HOCH-CH_2}{\underset{\displaystyle H_2C\quad CH}{|\quad\ \ |}}-COOH}}$$

Metabolism of aspartate, asparagine and alanine

COOH	Transamination	COOH
CH$_2$	⟶	CH$_2$
CH-NH$_2$		C = O
COOH		COOH
Aspartic acid		**Oxaloacetate**

NH$_2$		
C = O		COOH
CH$_2$	H$_2$O NH$_3$	CH$_2$
HC—NH$_2$	⟶	CH NH$_2$
COOH	Asparaginase	COOH
Asparagine		**Aspartic acid**

Asparaginase is used in acute lymphocytic leukemia, because leukemic cells require high concs of asparagine for their growth.

$$CH_3\underset{\underset{\displaystyle Alanine}{}}{-\underset{\overset{\displaystyle NH_2}{|}}{CH}-COOH} \xrightarrow[\text{Transamination}]{} CH_3\underset{\underset{\displaystyle Pyruvic\ acid}{}}{-\underset{\overset{\displaystyle O}{\|}}{C}-COOH}$$

Glycine, Serine and threonine metabolism

$$\underset{\underset{\displaystyle Serine}{}}{\underset{|}{\overset{OH}{}}\underset{|}{\overset{NH_2}{}}\!\!CH_2-CH-COOH} + THFA \rightleftharpoons NH_2-CH_2-COOH$$

Glycine

$$+ CH_2-THFA + H_2O$$

Serine   Tetrahydrofolic acid

Threonine is an essential amino acid Threonine is degraded in the body to give glycine and acetyl CoA Since glycine can be converted to 3-phosphoglycerate, threonine is glucogenic. The acetyl coA produced makes threonine also ketogenic.

Hormonal control of amino acid metabolism

Insulin and the somatomedins enhance the active transport of amino acids across cell membranes. Insulin inhibits gluconeogenesis from aminoacids and it promotes protein synthesis. Thyroid hormones also promote a positive nitrogen balance by stimulating protein synthesis. Glucocorticoids, like methylprednisolone, enhances gluconeogenesis from aminoacids. Therefore, high-dose glucocorticoid therapy leads to thinning of the skin and osteoporosis.

During fasting, the glucocorticoids predominate and insulin virtually disappears. The protein in skeletal muscle and in the viscera is lost daily by gluconeogenesis process to provide glucose.

Dietary carbohydrate is protein-sparing. At least 100 g of carbohydrate is required per day for adults to prevent excess protein catabolism via gluconeogenesis. Major quantity of the protein in a carbohydrate-deficient diet is not used for protein synthesis, instead, it enters gluconeogenesis to compensate for a lack of glucose. Therefore, the nitrogen balance is usually negative.

QUESTIONS

1. What are essential aminoacids, give examples for essential amino acids.
2. Define the term transamination. How it differs from deamination ?
3. How ammonia is removed from the body ?
4. What is meant by phenylketonuria ?
5. Write the biosynthesis of nor-adrenaline from phenylalanine.
6. Write the steps involved in the biosynthesis of cysteine.
7. What are the hormones which control the aminoacid metabolism?

9

CARBOHYDRATE METABOLISM

Human diet may contain carbohydrate in the form of polysaccharide (starch), disaccharide (sucrose, lactose) or monosaccharide (glucose, fructose, galactose).

Starch and other digestable carbohydrates are converted into monosaccharides by a series of hydrolytic enzyme. *Salivary amylase* (Ptyalin) is the enzyme present in saliva. It acts upon starch to hydrolyse it to maltose·Because the food is swallowed rapidly not much hydrolysis occurs in the mouth. However, the activity of the enzyme continues until the low pH of gastric juice inactivate it. About 40% hydrolysis occurs before inactivation by gastric acidity.

Pancreatic amylase (Amylopsin) splits starch and dextrin to maltose.

Pancreatic maltase catalyses the hydrolysis of maltose to glucose.

Intestinal lactase hydrolyses lactose to glucose and galactose

Intestinal maltase hydrolyses maltose to two molecules of glucose.

Intestinal sucrase hydrolyses sucrose to glucose and fructose.

ABSORPTION OF CARBOHYDRATES

Only monosaccharide are absorbed and can be utilised. The monosaccharides are absorbed at different rate into the blood stream. Suppose if the absorption of glucose is given a value of 100, the relative value for other monosaccharids are as follows.

D-galactose	110
D-Fructose	43
D-Mannose	19
D-xylose	15
D-Arabinose	9

After absorption they are carried by the portal circulation to the liver. In the liver, monosaccharides other than glucose are converted to glucose. This glucose may pass into general circulation or may be carried to tissues or may be converted to glycogen. This glycogen is the storage form of glucose. Glucose in tissue can be converted to muscle glycogen, which serves as a available source of energy for muscle. The lactic acid which results from glycogen breakdown is carried to liver where it is converted to liver glycogen. The above series of biotransformation is called Coricycle.

Biotransformation involved in carbohydrate metabolism

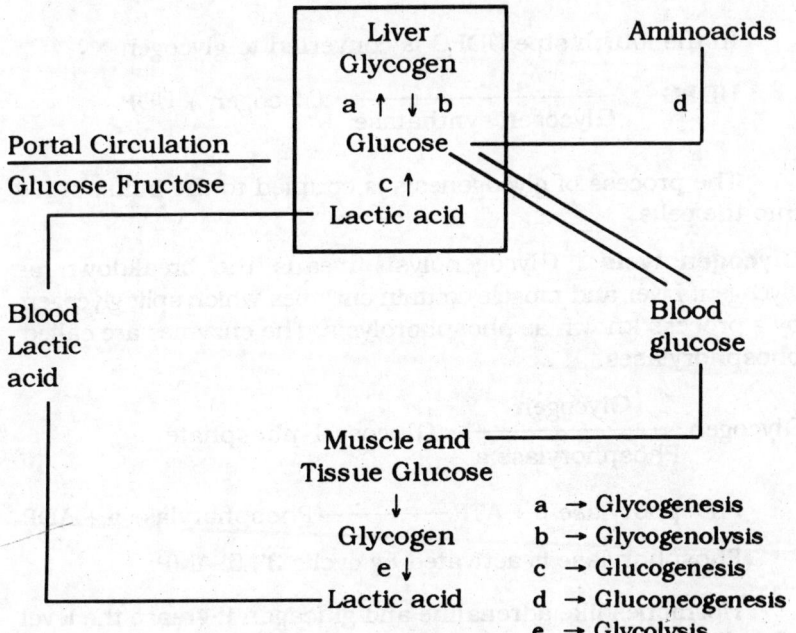

a	→ Glycogenesis
b	→ Glycogenolysis
c	→ Glucogenesis
d	→ Gluconeogenesis
e	→ Glycolysis

Glycogenesis : Glycogenesis means glycogen synthesis. Glycogene is the predominant polysaccharide present in the liver (upto 5-6%) and muscle (1%). It acts as a ready source of glucose units for maintenance of the blood glucose between meals. The first step in theglycogenesis process is the conversion of glucose to glucose 6-phosphate.

$$\text{Glucose} \xrightarrow[\substack{\text{Glucokinase} \\ \text{ATP Mg++ ADP}}]{} \text{Glucose 6-phosphate}$$

The above reaction is a phosphorylation reaction. In the second step glucose 6-phosphate is converted to Glucose 1-phosphate

$$\text{Glucose 6-phosphate} \xrightarrow[\substack{\text{Phosphoglucomutase} \\ \text{Mg++}}]{} \text{Glucose 1-phosphate}$$

In the third step Glucose 1-phosphate is converted to Uridine diphosphate glucose (UDPG)

$$\text{Glucose 1-phosphate} \xrightarrow[\text{UDPG pyrophosphorylase}]{\text{UTP} \rightarrow \text{PPi}} \text{UDPG}$$

In the fourth stpe UDPG is converted to glycogen

$$\text{UDPG} \xrightarrow[\text{Glycogen synthatase}]{} \text{Glycogen + UDP}$$

The process of glycogenesis is coupled to the influx of K+ into the cells.

Glycogenolysis : Glycogenolysis means the breakdown of glycogen. Liver and muscle contain enzymes which split glycogen by a process known as phosphorolysis. The enzymes are called phosphorylases.

$$\text{Glycogen} \xrightarrow[\substack{\text{Glycogen} \\ \text{Phosphorylase a}}]{} \text{Glucose 1-phosphate}$$

$$\text{Phsophorylase b + ATP} \longrightarrow \text{Phosphorylase a + ADP}$$

Phosphorylase is activated by cyclic 3', 5' AMP.

Hormones like adrenaline and glucagon increase the level of cyclic 3', 5' AMP and thus produce hyperglycemia. Where as insulin decreases the level of cyclic 3', 5' AMP and produces hypoglycemia.

$$\text{Glucose 1-phosphate} \xrightarrow{\text{Phosphoglucomutase}} \text{Glucose 6-phosphate}$$

$$\text{Glucose 6-Phosphate} \xrightarrow[\text{Glucose 6 phosphatase}]{\text{Liver}} \text{Glucose + Pi}$$

Glucose-6 phosphatase is absent in muscle.

The hereditary absence of muscle glycogen phosphorylase, termed type V glycogen storage disease (Mc Ardle's disease) causes glycogen to accumulate in skeletal muscle. During vigorous exercise glycogenolysis in muscle is impaired, causing muscle cramp and limited exercise tolerance.

Type III glycogen storage disease, the inherited deficiency of amylo-1, 6 glucosidase or oligo 1,4 → 1, 4 glucantransferase glucosidase in the liver and in heart and skeletal muscle, causes limit dextrins to accumulate in these tissues.

Glycolysis

The term glycolysis is restricted to a series of reaction involvedin biotransformation of glucose or glycogen to lactic acid. This series of reaction is known as Embden-Meyer-hof pathway. In the presence of oxygen pyruvate is formed as the end product instead of lactic acid.

The enzymes for glycolysis are found in the extramitochondrial fraction of the cell. The steps and enzymes involved in glycolysis are as follows :

$$\alpha\text{-D-Glucose} \xrightarrow[\underset{\text{ATP ADP}}{\text{Hexokinase}}]{\text{Mg}^{++}} \alpha\text{-D-Glucose 6-phosphate} \xrightarrow[\text{isomerase}]{\substack{\text{Glucose} \\ \text{Phosphate}}} \text{D-fructose 6-phosphate}$$

$$\text{ADP} \leftarrow \text{ATP} \quad \underset{\text{Mg}^{++}}{\text{Phosphofructokinase}}$$

D-Fructose 1,6-diphosphate

2 moles 1,3-diphospho-glycerate ← NADH + H NAD 2 mole of Glyceral--dehyde 3-phosphate ← Dehydrogenase ←→ isomer--ase ← Aldolase → Dihydroxyacetone phosphate

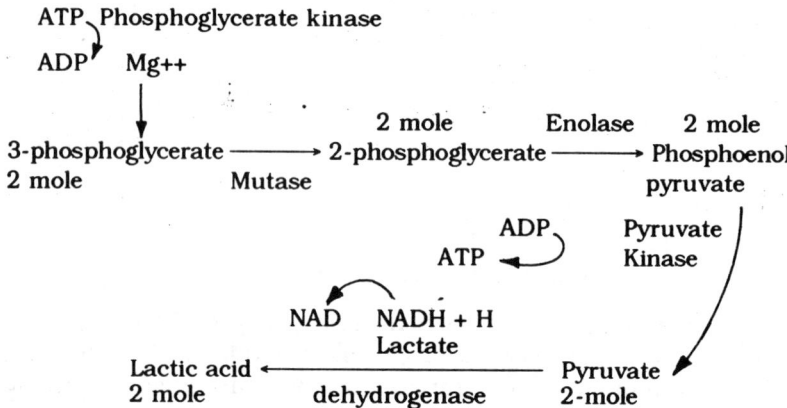

In tissues with adequate oxygen supply, pyruvate formation is the last step of glycolysis. Most of this pyruvate undergoes oxidative decarboxylation to form an acetyl CoA mole, which enters the tricarboxylic acid cycle.

Anaerobic tissues, such as exercising muscle or in cases of coronary artery disease, an inadequately perfused myocardium, cannot utilize the Krebs cycle or oxidative phosphorylation. Hence, NADH produced by the glyceraldehydephosphate dehydrogenase reaction accumulates, while NAD becomes scarce. However, the lactate dehydrogenase uses NADH to reduce pyruvate to lactate.

$$
\begin{array}{ccc}
\underset{|}{COOH} & & \underset{|}{COOH} \\
\underset{|}{C = 0} & \text{LDH} & \underset{|}{HC - OH} \\
CH_3 & +NADH + H \longrightarrow & CH_3 \\
\text{Pyruvate} & & \text{Lactic acid}
\end{array}
$$

Lactic acid diffuses into the bloodstream and reaches the liver, where it is oxidized back to pyruvate.

Citric acid cycle (Krebs cycle, Tricarboxylic acid cycle)

When the glycolysis process occurs in the anaerobic condition pyruvate is reduced to lactate.

But in aerobic condition the electrons are transferred through the electron transport system maintaining the NAD in the oxidised form. Under these conditions pyruvate is not reduced to lactate but is further oxidised to carbon dioxide and water through the Krebs cycle. The enzymes for the Krebs cycle are present in the mitochondrial fraction of the cell. Krebs cycle provides most of the energy for the endergonic process. It also acts as a common pathway for the oxidation of carbohydrates, protein and lipids.

It also plays a major role in gluconeogenesis, transamination and lipogenesis process. Liver is the major organ where these reactions takes place.

The steps involved in Kerbs cycle are as follows :

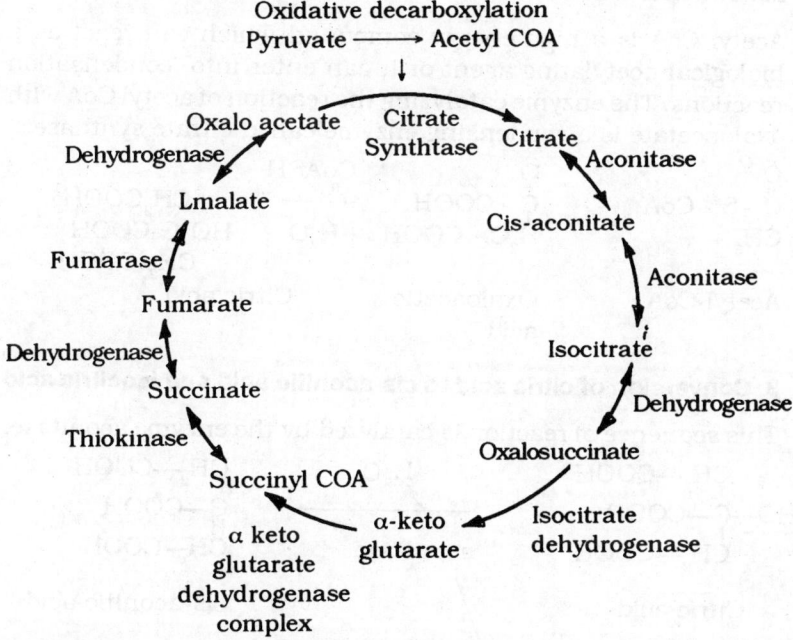

Total 38 mole cules of ATP are formed from one molecule of glucose under aerobic oxidation.

INDIVIDUAL REACTIONS OF CITRIC ACID CYCLE

1. Formation of acetyl COA

Pyruvic acid is activated before entering into Krebs cycle by forming acetyl COA.

$$\begin{array}{c} COOH \\ | \\ C = O \\ | \\ CH_3 \end{array} + CoASH \xrightarrow[\text{NAD \quad NADH + H}]{\overset{\textstyle Mg^{++}}{\text{TPP, Lipoic acid}}} \begin{array}{c} O \\ \| \\ C-S-CoA \\ | \\ CH_3 + CO_2 \end{array}$$

Pyruvic acid	Pyruvate Dehydrogenase Complex	Acetyl COA

The major source of acetyl COA is from the oxidation of carbohydrates or fatty acids.

2. Formation of citric acid

Acetyl CoA is a high energy compound which can react as a biological acetylating agent or it can enter into condensation reactions. The enzyme catalyzing the reaction of acetyl CoA with oxaloacetate is a condensing enzyme called citrate synthase

$$\begin{array}{c} O \\ \| \\ C - S - CoA \\ | \\ CH_3 \end{array} + \begin{array}{c} O \\ \| \\ C - COOH \\ | \\ H_2C - COOH \end{array} + H_2O \xrightarrow{\text{CoASH}} \begin{array}{c} CH_2COOH \\ | \\ HO-C-COOH \\ | \\ CH_2-COOH \end{array}$$

Acetyl CoA	Oxaloacetic acid	Citric acid

3. Conversion of citric acid to cis-aconitic acid and isocitric acid

This sequence of reaction is catalyzed by the enzyme aconitase.

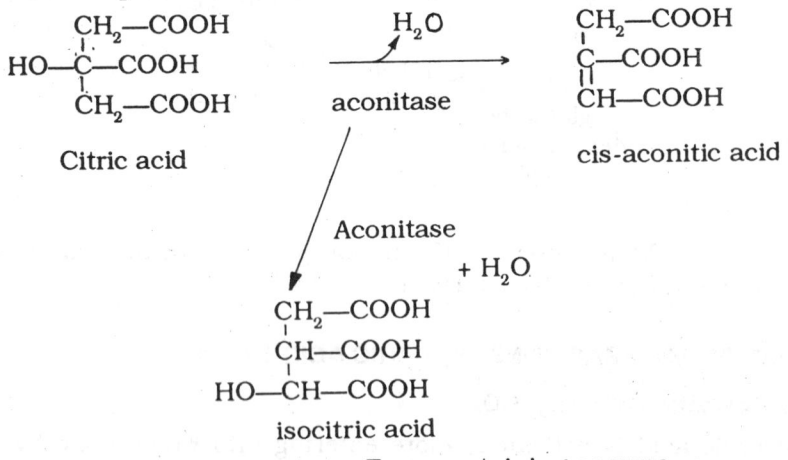

Aconitase is an Fe++ containing enzyme.

4. Formation of α-ketoglutaric acid

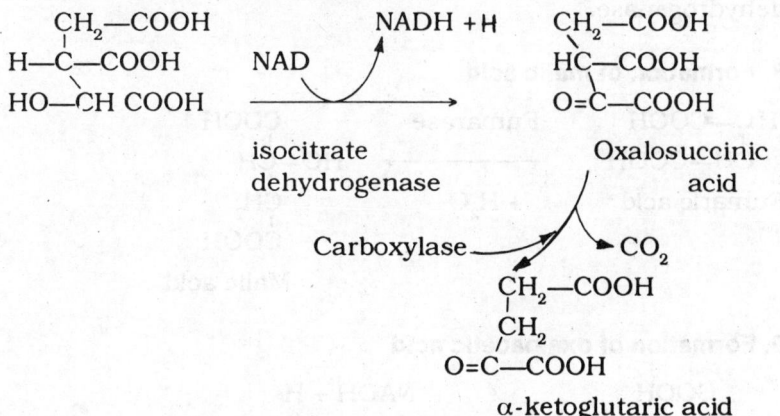

α-ketoglutaric acid

5. Oxidative-decarboxylation of α-ketoglutarate

CH₂—COOH
CH₂   TPP, Mg++, Lipoic acid   CH₂—COOH
C = O + CoASH   ——————————————→   CH₂
COOH   NAD   NADH + H   O=C+CO₂
                                                S – CoA

α-ketoglutaric   Succinyl CoA
acid

This reaction is not reversible and this irreversibility prevents the Krebs cycle from running in the reverse direction.

6. Conversion of succinyl CoA to succinic acid

CH₂—COOH
CH₂   Thiokinase   CH₂—COOH
C = O   ——————————————→   CH₂—COOH   + COASH
S—CoA   Pi + GDP GTP   Succinic acid

Succinyl CoA

7. Conversion of succinic acid to fumaric acid

CH₂ - COOH   Succinate dehydrogenase   CH—COOH
CH₂ - COOH   ——————————————→   HOOC—CH
                      FAD FADH₂   Fumaric acid

Malonic acid is a competitive inhibitor of succinic dehydrogenase.

8. Formation of malic acid

$$
\begin{array}{lll}
\underset{\text{Fumaric acid}}{\overset{\displaystyle \text{HC—COOH}}{\underset{\displaystyle \text{CH—COOH}}{\|}}} &
\underset{+\ H_2O}{\text{Fumarase} \longrightarrow} &
\underset{\text{Malic acid}}{\overset{\displaystyle \text{COOH}}{\underset{\displaystyle \overset{\displaystyle \text{HO—CH}}{\underset{\displaystyle \text{COOH}}{\text{CH}_2}}}{|}}}
\end{array}
$$

9. Formation of oxaloacetic acid

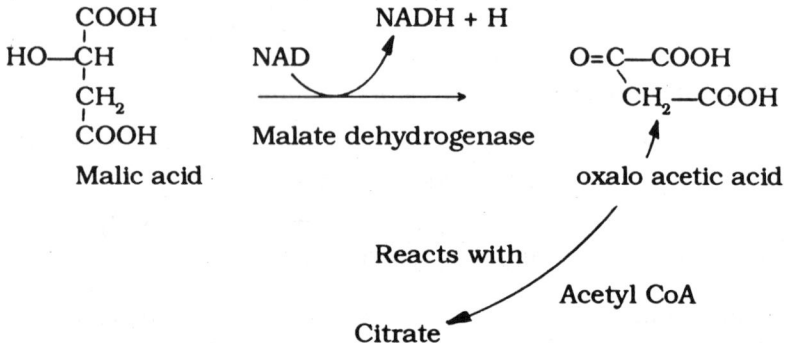

In carbohydrate deficiency, there is not enough pyruvate for the pyruvate carboxylase reaction, which causes depletion of TCA - cycle intermediates and excess fat mobilization.

OXIDATION AND REDUCTION REACTIONS

Oxidation and reduction reactions take place in the body. During the oxidation oxygen is consumed and carbondioxide is produced.

$$\text{FOOD} + O_2 \longrightarrow CO_2 + H_2O$$

During the oxidation process the body get a lot of energy.

Oxidation are 3 types

1. Addition of oxygen to a molecule

e.g. $\underset{\text{Acetaldehyde}}{CH_3—CHO} \longrightarrow \underset{\text{Acetic acid}}{CH_3\ COOH}$

2. Removal of hydrogen from a molecule

e.g. $CH_3-CH_2-OH \longrightarrow CH_3-CHO + H_2$
       Alcohol   Acetaldehyde

3. Loss of an electron

e.g. $Fe^{++} \longrightarrow Fe^{+++} + e$

ANAEROBIC OXIDATION

In case of anaerobic oxidation, the oxidation takes place without the involvement of oxygen. Here other substances act as hydrogen acceptor. The hydrogen acceptors may be Nicotinamide adenine dinucleotide (NAD), Nicotinamide adenine dinucleotide phosphate (NADP), Cytochrome and Flavin adenine dinucleotide (FAD).

e.g. NAD is required for the oxidation of lactate to pyruvate

NADP is essential for the oxidation of Glucose - 6 - phosphate to 6-phosphogluconate. FAD is required for the conversion of succinic acid to fumaric acid

Ubiquinone (coenzyme Q)

It is a hydrogen acceptor present in mitochondria.

Cytochromes

Cytochromes are mixture of haemochromogen like compounds present in all oxygen utilizing tissues. Iron is present in all oxygen utilizing tissues. Iron is present in Fe^{++} and Fe^{+++} form in the cytochrome. This property is useful for the transfer of electron from reduced flavoprotein to oxygen.

$$2Fe^{+++} + RH_2 \longrightarrow R + 2Fe^{++} + 2H$$
$$2Fe^{++} + O + 2H \longrightarrow 2\,Fe^{+++} + H_2O$$

Five components of cytochrome system are cytochrome a, cytochrome a_3, cytochrome b, cytochrome c and cytochrome c_1. Cytochrome a_3 is the final catalyst in the oxidation system.

Aerobic oxidation

In this type of oxidation molecular oxygen is the hydrogen

acceptor

$$XH_2 + O \xrightarrow{\text{oxidase}} X + H_2O$$

$$XH_2 + O_2 \xrightarrow[\text{dehydrogenase}]{\text{aerobic}} X + H_2O_2$$

Aerobic oxidases are metalloprotein e.g. cytochrome oxidase, ascorbic oxidase, tyrosinase, uricase, phenol oxidase etc.

The Electron Transport system

When a molecule of glucose is processed through the reactions of glycolysis and the citric acid cycle, its hydrogen atoms are removed. It is well known the when hydrogen and oxygen combine, much energy is released. When liberated too suddenly, the energy of hydrogen is difficult to handle. The cell guards against the problem and liberating its energy in a series of steps by a special mechanism called the *electron transporrt system*.

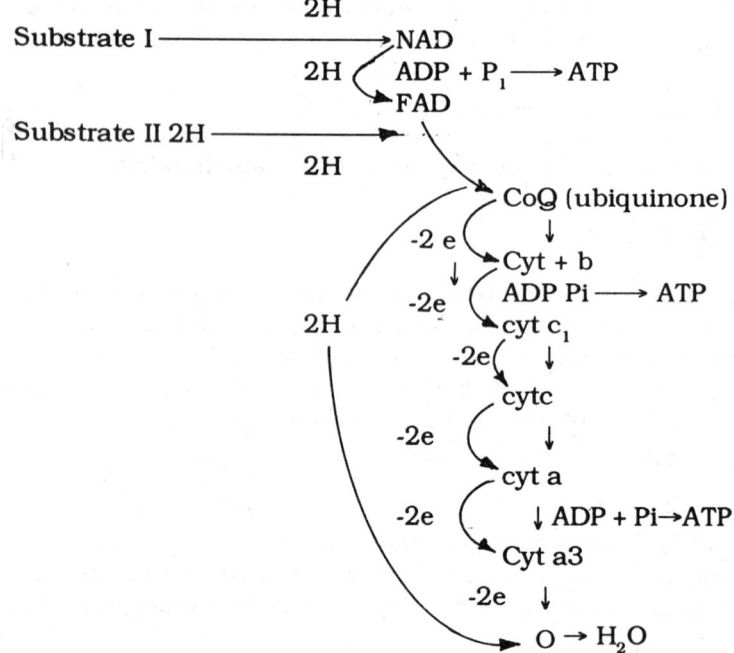

Initially the hydrogen is accepted by a compound called nicotinamide adenine dinucleotide (NAD) By accepting hydrogen, it becomes $NADH_2$. Hydrogen is then passed on to a second compound called flavin adenine dinucleotide (FAD). When FAD accepts hydrogen it becomes $FADH_2$. Here, the hydrogen loss (or electron loss) counts as oxidation and hydrogen acceptance (or electron acceptance) as reduction. Electron is passed from one electron acceptor to another. These electron acceptors are pigments called cytochromes. At two points inthe cytochrome system there is enough potential energy difference to produce ATP. In the end these electrons, now almost drained of energy by the cytochrome oxidase system, are accepted by oxygen with no more than a slight production of warmth. The protons, too, head for the oxygen, and upon reaching it reconstitute the two hydrogens, not as hydrogen but as part of water. For every two hydrogen atoms that pass through the electron transport system three ATPs are produced.

Aerobic versus anaerobic respiration

More than 90% of ATP formed in most cell is produced via aerobic respiration. 38 molecules of ATP can be produced from each glucose molecule that is completely oxidized.

When sufficient oxygen is not available to receive the hydrogens passed down the electron transport system, the last cytochrome in the chain is stuck with the hydrogen. The preceding carrier molecule then has no acceptor to which to give its hydrogen electrons, and the entire system becomes blocked all the way back to NAD. No further ATP can be produced by way of the electron transport system. Most cells cannot live long without oxygen because the amount of energy that can be produced anaerobically is not sufficient to sustain life.

Comparison of anaerobic with aerobic pathway is given below :

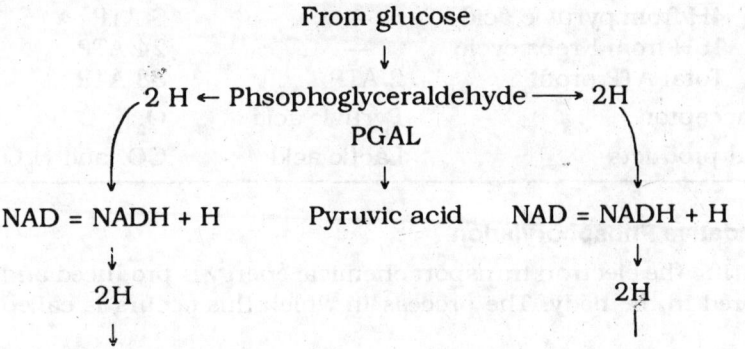

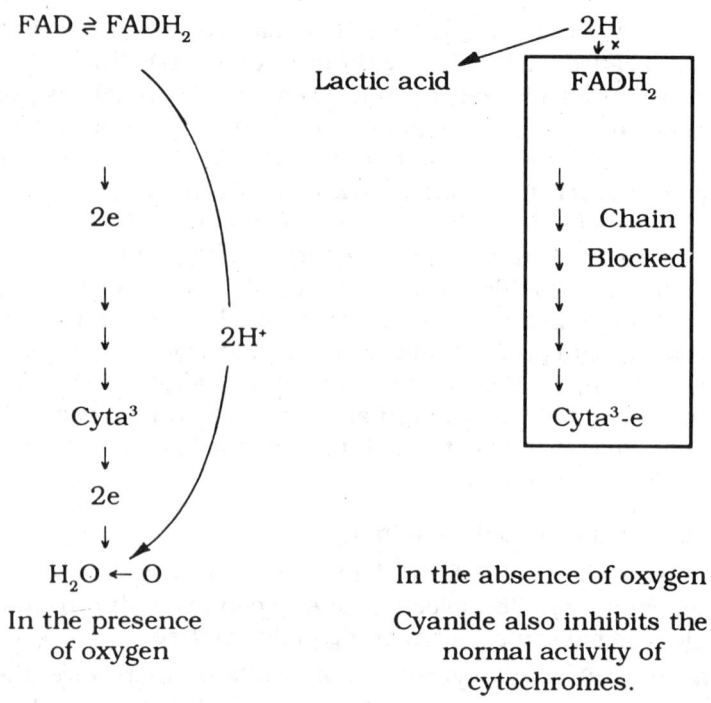

In the presence of oxygen

In the absence of oxygen

Cyanide also inhibits the normal activity of cytochromes.

The following table shows the generation of ATP molecules from *glucose* during aerobic and anaerobic respiration

	Anaerobic	**Aerobic**
ATP profit (gain) from Glycolysis	2ATP	2ATP
By way of electron transport systtem		
4H from glycolysis	—	6 ATP
4H from pyruvic acid	—	6 ATP
16H from Krebs cycle	—	24 ATP
Total ATP profit	2 ATP	38 ATP
H acceptor	Pyruvic acid	O_2
End products	Lactic acid	CO_2 and H_2O

Oxidative Phosphorylation

During the electron transport chemical energy is produced and stored in the body. The process in which this occurs is called oxidative phosphorylation because oxidation and phosphorylation reactions are involved in the production ATP molecules.

GLUCONEOGENESIS

Gluconeo genesis is a process by which glucose or glycogen are formed from non-carbohydrate source.

The steps involved in gluconeogenesis process are as follows :

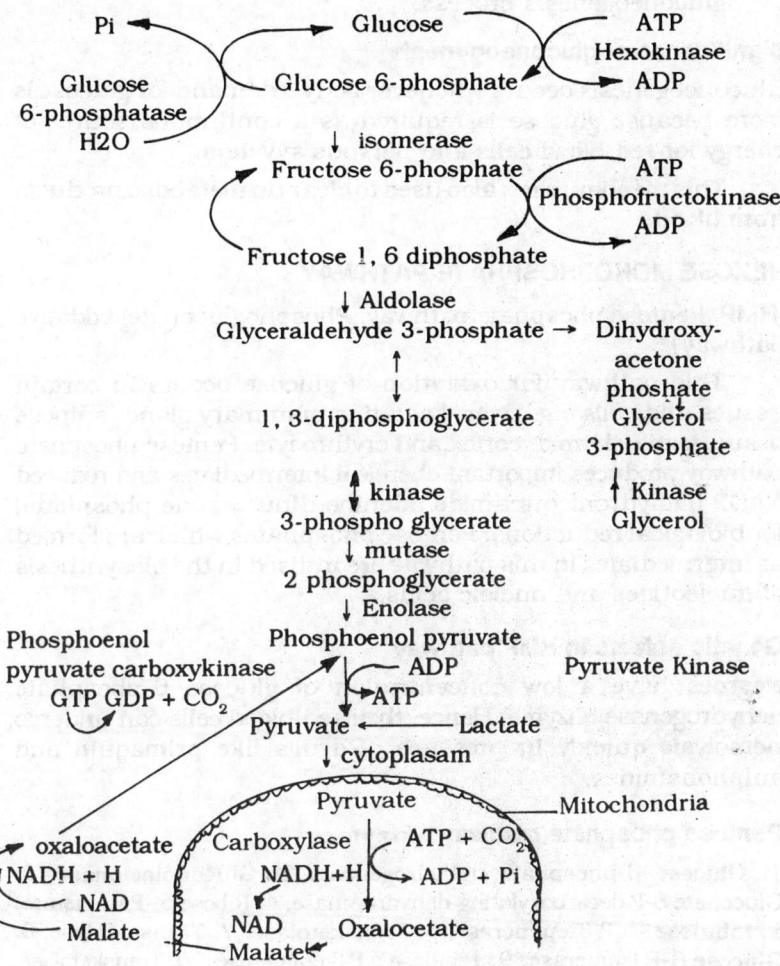

Substrate for gluconeogenesis

(a) Glucogenic aminoacids (Antiketogenic amino acids) Glycine, Alanin, Serine, Cystine, valine, Aspartate, Arginine, Proline, Hydroxyproline.
These aminoacids are deaminated to form ketoacids. From these ketoacids glucose is formed.

(b) Lactic acid

(c) Glycerol
Liver and kidney are the organs responsible for gluconeogenesis process.

Significance of gluconeogenesis

Gluconeogenesis occurs whenever body's demand for glucose is more because glucose is required as a continuous source of energy for red blood cells and nervous syystem.

This mechanism is also used to clear up metabolic products from blood.

HEXOSE MONOPHOSPHATE PATHWAY

(HMP, Pentose phosphate pathway, Phosphogluconate oxidative pathway)

This pathway for oxidation of glucose occurs in certain tissues and cells e.g. Liver, Lactating mammary gland, adipose tissue, testis, thyroid, cortex and erythrocyte. Pentose phosphate pathway produces important chemical intermediates and reduced NADP (Dihydronicotinamide adenine dinucleotide phosphate) for biological reductions. Pentose phosphates which are formed as intermediates in this pathway are utilised in the biosynthesis of nucleotides and nucleic acids.

Genetic defects in HMP pathway

Negroes have a low concentration of glucose 6-phosphate dehydrogenase enzyme. Hence, their red blood cells can undergo hemolysis quickly in presence of drugs like primaquin and sulphonamides.

Pentose phosphate pathway Enzymes

1. Glucose 6-phosphate dehydrogenase, 2. Gluconolactonase, 3. Gluconate 6-P decarboxylating-dehydrogenase, 4. Ribose 5 -P isomerase, 5. Ribulose -5 P 3-epimerase, 6. Transketolase, 7. Transaldolase, 8. Glucose 6-P isomerase, 9. Ribulose 5 P 3 epimerase, 10. Transketolase, 11. Glucose 6 P isomerase, 12. Aldolase, 13. Fructose 1 : 6 di P - 1 - P hydrolase, 14. Glucose 6-P isomerase

Pentose phosphate pathway

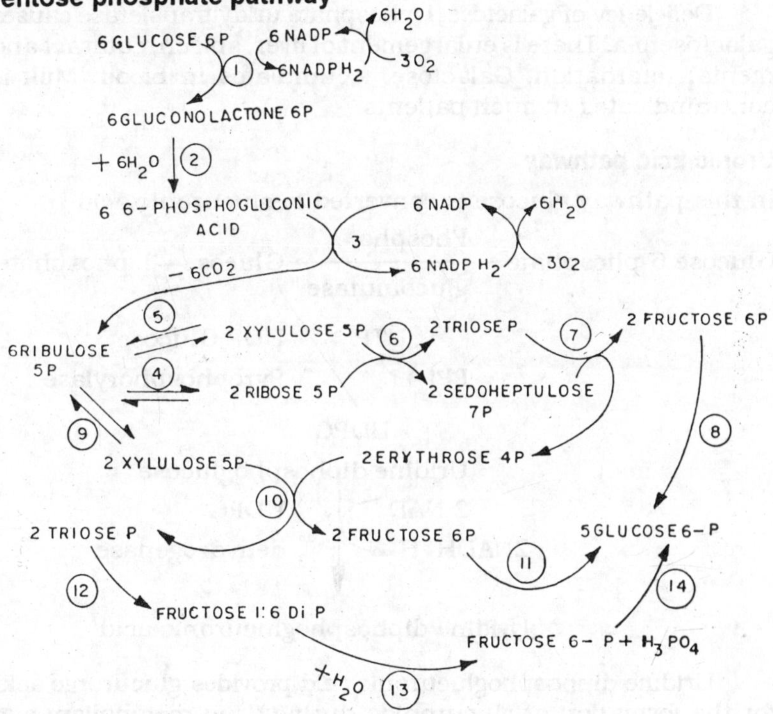

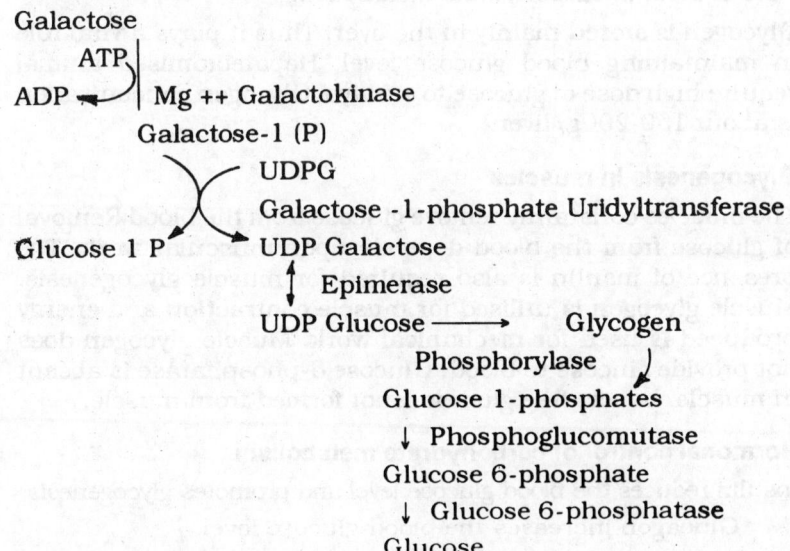

Metabolism of galactose

Galactose

ATP
ADP ⟶| Mg ++ Galactokinase

Galactose-1 (P)

UDPG

Galactose -1-phosphate Uridyltransferase

Glucose 1 P   UDP Galactose

↕ Epimerase

UDP Glucose ⟶ Glycogen

Phosphorylase

Glucose 1-phosphates

↓ Phosphoglucomutase

Glucose 6-phosphate

↓ Glucose 6-phosphatase

Glucose

Deficiency of galactose-1-phosphate uridyltransferase causes galactosemia. There is enlargement of liver, spleen, cataract and mental retardation. Galactose accumulates in blood. Milk is contraindicated in such patients.

Uronic acid pathway

In this pathway glucose is converted to glucuronic acid

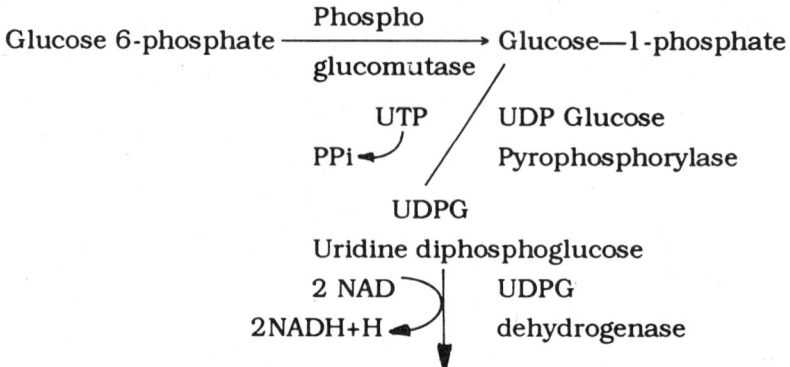

Uridine diphosphoglucuronic acid provides glucuronic acid for the formation of glucuronide during drug metabolism e.g. Paracetamol is converted in the body to a glucuronide.

Role of Liver in carbohydrate metabolism

Glycogen is stored mainly in the liver. Thus it plays a vital role in maintaining blood glucose level. Hepatectomised animal require high dose of glucose to survive. Glycogen concentration is about 150-200g/liver.

Glycogenesis in muscles

The muscles constantly remove glucose from the blood. Removal of glucose from the blood depends upon muscular work. The presence of insulin is also required for muscle glycogenesis. Muscle glycogen is utilised for muscle contraction and energy produced is used for mechanical work. Muscle glycogen does not provide glucose to blood. Glucose 6-phosphatase is absent in muscle, hence, free glucose isnot formed from muscle.

Hormonal control of carbohydrate metabolism

Insulin reduces the blood glucose level and promotes glycogenesis.

Glucagon increases the blood glucose level.

Adrenaline and glucocorticoids also increase the blood glucose level.

Carbohydrate tolerance : It is the ability of the body to utilize glucose.

Carbohydrate tolerance is less under the following conditions.

(a) Lack of insulin (Diabetes mellitus)

(b) Liver damage

(c) Atherosclerosis

(e) Hyperactivity of pituitary

(f) Hyperactivity of adrenal cortex.

The tolerance increases during the following conditions

(a) In presence of insulin

(b) Hypopituitarism

(c) Adrenocortical insufficiency

Glucose Tolerance Test

Glucose tolerance test depends upon the blood and urine sugar determination. Fasting blood and urine samples are collected and the patient is given 75-100 grams of glucose dissolved in 400 ml of water (Zero hour).

Four morre samples of blood and Urine are collected after every half an hour after the administration of glucose. All the samples are analysed for their glucose contents. A graph is plotted by taking time in minutes on the x-axis and mg% glucose on the Y-axis as shown below.

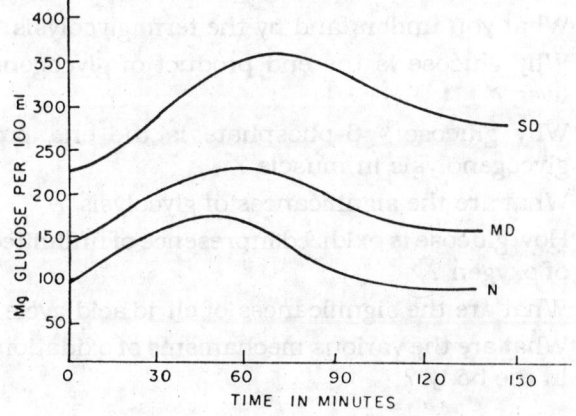

In a normal person the fasting blood sugar level is between 80-120 mg%.

In mild diabetes (curve (MD) the fasting blood sugar levl is slightly higher than 120 mg%. In severe diabetes (SD) the fasting blood sugar level is higher than 200 mg%.

Incase of severe diabetes the blood glucose level rises rapidly after the ingestion of glucose and does not come down significantly at the end of two hours,Sugar is also present in the fasting urine sample.

Renal diabetes

Here the blood glucose levels are normal but sugar appears in urine. This is due to very low kidney threshold for glucose.

QUESTIONS

1. What is the funtion of salivary amylase ?
2. How carbohydrates are digested in the intestine ?
3. Which monosaccharide is absorbed fast into the blood stream ?
4. What is coricycle ?
5. Define the term glycogenesis
6. Name the major sites where glycogne is stored.
7. What is glycogenolysis ?
8. Which is the active form of phosphorylase enzyme ?
9. What is Mc Ardle's disease ?
10. What you understand by the term glycolysis ?
11. Why glucose is the end product of glycogenolysis in liver ?
12. Why glucose - 6-phosphate is the end product of glycogenolysis in muscle ?
13. What are the significances of glycolysis ?
14. How glucose is oxidized inpresence of unlimited supply of oxygen ?
15. What are the significances of citric acid cycle ?
16. What are the various mechanisms of oxidation process in the body ?

17. What do you understand by the term Electron Transport System ?
18. What is meant by oxidative phosphorylation ?
19. What is gluconeogenesis ?
20. What are glucogenic amino acids ?
21. Where does citric acid cycle occur in the cell ?
22. What are the significance of hexose monophosphate shunt pathway ?
23. What is galactosemia ?
24. What do you understand by uronic acid pathway ?
25. What is meant by glucose tolerance ? Name the conditions which modify glucose tolerance.
26. What is glucose tolerance test ?
27. What is renal diabetes ?

10

METABOLISM OF LIPIDS

Lipids are esters of fatty acids with glycerol. Lipids are important component along with other food material. During digestion lipids are hydrolysed by lipases and phosphatases to fatty acid, glycerol, phosphoric acid and other products.

GASTRIC DIGESTION

There is no digestion of fat in the mouth. Gastric lipase is inhibited by gastric acidity, because of this there is little splitting of fat. in the stomach. But if excess of fats are taken then regurgitation may occur. Thus pancreatic lipase may enter the stomach.

Intestinal digestion

In the small intestine fat is hydrolysed by pancreatic lipase. As such pancreatic lipase is inactive and is activated by calcium salt and bile salts. Bile salts are essential for emulsification of fat. Soluble proteins also help in the emulsification and absorption of fatty acid. Intestinal juice also contains lipase which can act upon any fat unaffected by pancreatic lipase.

Absorption of Lipids

Partially hydrolysed lipid is readily absorbed in the last portion of duodenum and proximal part of jejunum. Lipids are also absorbed by pinocytosis process, lipids pass through the membrane by diffusion.

Passage of the absorbed lipids into the blood

Lipids, whether absorbed as such or re-synthesized in the epithelial cell enter the lymphatic vessels as a milky emulsion called chyle. The minute droplets of fat are chylomicron. Chylomicron consists of triglycerides, phospholipid, free fatty acid and they are surrounded by thin layer of protein. These particles passes through lymphatic duct of abdominal cavity and then enters into blood through the thoracic duct.

Oxidation of fatty acids

Oxidation of fatty acids provides high energy to the tissues (9 k cal g^{-1})

Sources of fatty acids

(a) Mammalian tissue contain only very small quantity of free fatty acids.
(b) Fatty acids are formed from the hydrolysis of triglycerides due to the action of hormonally controlled lipase.
(c) The released free fatty acid from tissue is bound to serum albumin of the blood and is taken to various parts of the tissue for oxidation.

Tissues involved in the oxidation of long chain fatty acid

Liver, kidney, heartmuscle, lungs, testis and adipose tissue.

The pathway of fatty acid oxidation

Fatty acids undergo β-oxidation inside the cell at the mitochondrial site. Carnitine helps in the transport of acylco-A from the extramitochondrial part to mitochondrial site.

$$R-CH_2-CH_2-\underset{\underset{O}{\|}}{C}-OH \qquad \text{Fatty acid}$$

COASH

Thiokinase

ATP Mg++

AMP+PPi

Cytoplasm

- -

Mitochondria

$$R-CH_2-CH_2-\underset{\underset{O}{\|}}{C}\sim S-CoA \qquad \text{Acyl CoA}$$

Acyl CoA
dehydrogenase $\overset{\displaystyle \curvearrowright FAD}{\displaystyle \leftarrow FADH+H}$

$$R—CH=CH—\underset{\underset{O}{||}}{C}{\sim}S—CoA$$ α, β unsaturated
Acyl CoA

Δ^2 Enoyl CoA
hydratase $\quad \overset{\curvearrowright H_2O}{\downarrow}$

$$\underset{\underset{O}{||}}{\overset{\overset{OH}{|}}{R—CH—CH_2—C}}{\sim}S—CoA$$ β-Hydroxy acyl Co A

Dehydrogenase $\overset{\curvearrowright NAD}{\underset{\curvearrowleft NADH+H}{\downarrow}}$

$$R—\underset{\underset{O}{||}}{C}—CH_2—\underset{\underset{O}{||}}{C}—S—CoA$$ β-Ketoacylco A

β-ketothiolase $\quad \overset{\curvearrowright CoASH}{\downarrow}$

$$R—\underset{\underset{O}{||}}{C}{\sim}S—CoA + CH_3—\underset{\underset{O}{||}}{C}{\sim}S—CoA$$

Acyl CoA $\qquad\qquad$ Acetyl CoA
$\qquad\qquad\qquad\qquad\qquad\downarrow$
$\qquad\qquad\qquad\qquad$ Krebscycle

Oxidation of Odd-Carbon Fatty Acids and the fate of Propionyl CoA

These are rare in human system, however, they occur in some marine organism. The odd carbon fatty acid undergo similar type of reaction (i.e. β-oxidation). the end product formed is propionyl-CoA instead of acetyl CoA. This propionyl CoA is converted to succinyl CoA.

$$CH_3—CH_2—\underset{\underset{O}{||}}{C}—OH \xrightarrow[\substack{ATP \\ CoASH}]{\overset{\text{Thiokinase}}{\quad\quad\quad}\; {}^{\displaystyle\searrow AMP+PP}} CH_3—CH_2—\underset{\underset{O}{||}}{C}—S—CoA$$

Propionic acid $\qquad\qquad\qquad\qquad\qquad\qquad$ Propionyl CoA

$\qquad\qquad\qquad\qquad$ Biotin CO_2 $\overset{\curvearrowright ATP}{\underset{\searrow ADP}{\Big|}}$
$\qquad\qquad\qquad\qquad$ Carboxy- Co_2+
$\qquad\qquad\qquad\qquad$ lase, H_2O

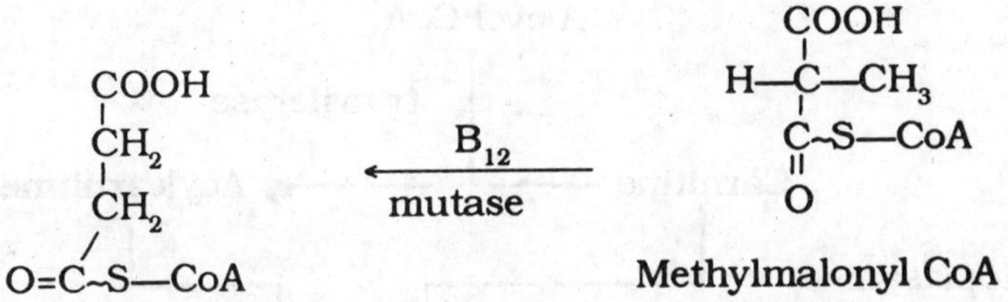

$$\text{Succinyl CoA} \xleftarrow[\text{mutase}]{B_{12}} \text{Methylmalonyl CoA} + ADP + Pi$$

```
        COOH                              COOH
        |                                 |
        CH₂              B₁₂          H—C—CH₃
        |          ←————————              |
        CH₂            mutase          C~S—CoA
        /                              ‖
   O=C~S—CoA                           O
   Succinyl CoA                    Methylmalonyl CoA
        |                             +ADP+Pi
        ↓
   Krebs cycle
```

Oxidation of Unsaturated fatty acid

Unsaturated fatty acids (Oleic, linoleic, linolenic and arachidonic) are oxidised in the same way as β-oxidation. But the double bond which are in cis Configuration are first converted into trans form by isomerase enzyme and hydratase enzyme and then converted to acetyl CoA.

e.g.

$$\text{Linoleyl CoA}$$
$$\downarrow$$
$$\Delta^3 \text{ cis-}\Delta^6 \text{cis dienonyl CoA}$$
$$\downarrow \quad \text{Enoyl CoA isomerase}$$
$$\Delta^2 \text{ trans } \Delta^6 \text{ cis Dienonyl CoA}$$
$$\downarrow \quad \text{Hydratase}$$
$$\beta\text{-hydroxyacyl CoA}$$
$$\downarrow$$
$$\text{Acetyl CoA.}$$

ROLE OF CARNITINE IN FATTY ACID METABOLISM

Carnitine is present in muscle

It stimulates the oxidation of long chain fatty acids in mitochondria. The long chain fatty acids in the form of acyl CoA will not penetrate into mitochondria unless carnitine is present.

The mechanism by which carnitine promotes the β-oxidation is shown below.

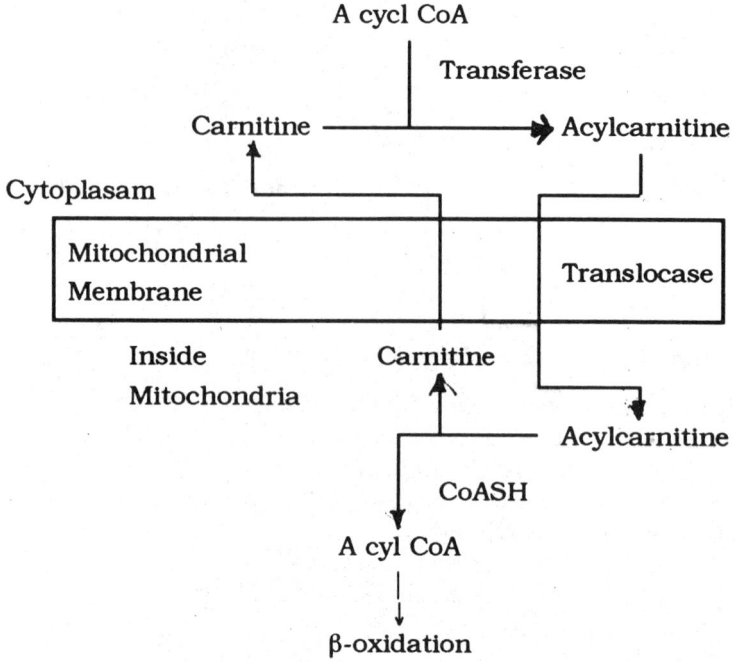

ESSENTIAL FATTY ACIDS

Linoleic acid
Linolenic acid
Arachidonic acid

These fatty acids are called as essential fatty acids because body cannot synthesize these acids. These acids are required to maintain good health. Unsaturated fatty acids also under go β-oxidation reaction in the mitochondria.

Functions of essential free fatty acids

(a) They are present in the structural lipids of the cell.

(b) They are present in the mitochondrial membrane.

(c) High concentration of essential fatty acid required for the reproductive function.

Synthesis of fatty acid

Synthesis of fatty acid takes palce in two sites of the cell.

(a) Mitochondria

(b) Extyramitochondiral region.

In the mitochondria already exsisting short chain fatty acid will be extended.

Synthesis of fatty acids at Extramitochondrial system

It occurs mainly in tissues like liver, kidney, brain lung, mammary gland and adipose tissue.

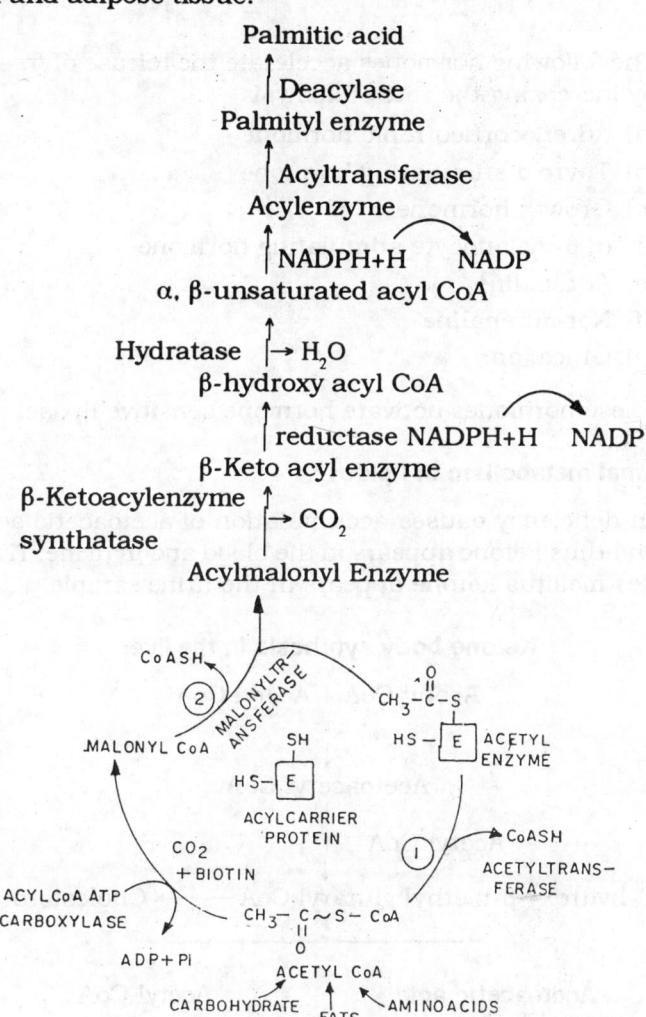

Palmitic acid

↑ Deacylase

Palmityl enzyme

↑ Acyltransferase

Acylenzyme

↑ NADPH+H ⟶ NADP

α, β-unsaturated acyl CoA

↑

Hydratase ⊢→ H_2O

β-hydroxy acyl CoA

↑ reductase NADPH+H ⟶ NADP

β-Keto acyl enzyme

β-Ketoacylenzyme ↑

synthatase ⊢→ CO_2

Acylmalonyl Enzyme

Influence of hormones on fat metabolism in adipose tissue

Insulin : Insulin reduces plasma free fatty acid. It inhibits the release of free fatty acid.

Insulin promotes lipogenesis. It increases the utilization of glucose in adipose tissue. It inhibits the hormone sensitive lipase.

The following hormones accelerate the release of free fatty acid by increasing the rate of lipolysis

(a) Adrenocorticotropic hormone

(b) Thyroid stimulating hormone

(c) Growth hormone

(d) α, β-melanocyte stimulating hormone

(e) Adrenaline

(f) Nor-adrenaline

(g) Glucagon

These hormones activate hormone sensitive lipase.

Abnormal metabolism of lipids

Insulin deficiency causes accumulation of acetoacetic acid in liver and thus ketone appears in the blood and in urine. Thus in diabetes mellitus ketone appears in the urine sample.

Ketone body synthesis in the liver

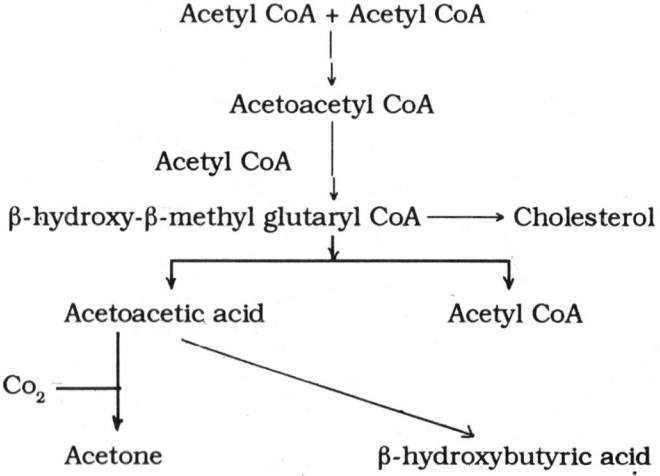

High concentration of β-hydroxy-β-methyl glutaryl CoA leads to the excess synthesis of cholesterol and its deposit on blood vessels. Hyperlipidemia and altherosclerosis occurs.

Ketone-body degradation in extrahepatic tissues

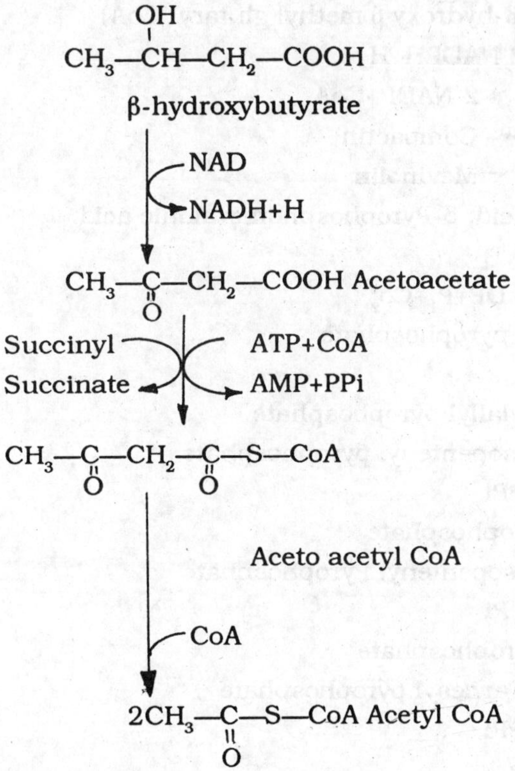

$$OH$$
$$CH_3—CH—CH_2—COOH$$

β-hydroxybutyrate

NAD

NADH+H

$$CH_3—C—CH_2—COOH \text{ Acetoacetate}$$
$$O$$

Succinyl — ATP+CoA

Succinate — AMP+PPi

$$CH_3—C—CH_2—C—S—CoA$$
$$O \qquad O$$

Aceto acetyl CoA

CoA

$$2CH_3—C—S—CoA \text{ Acetyl CoA}$$
$$O$$

Cholesterol biosynthesis

Human body has two sources of cholesterol :

(i) Diets

(i) Synthesis from acetate.

The greater the dietary intake of cholesterol, the lower the rate of cholesterol biosynthesis in the liver and adrenal cortex.

Tissues involved in the biosynthesis of cholesterol are liver, adrenal cortex, skin, intestine, testis and aorta.

Steps involved in the biosynthesis of cholesterol are :

2 Acetyl CoA

$\longrightarrow$ CoA

Acetoacetyl CoA

$\longrightarrow$ Acetyl CoA

$\longrightarrow$ CoA

HMG-CoA (β-hydroxy β methyl glutaryl CoA)

Reductase $\mid$ 2 NADPH+H

$\searrow$ 2 NADP+CoA

$\longleftarrow$ Compactin

$\longleftarrow$ Mevinolin

Mevalonic acid, 5-Pyrophosphomevalonic acid

ATP

$\downarrow$ $\searrow$ ADP+P_1+CO_2

Isopentenyl pyrophosphate

$\downarrow$

3,3-dimethylallyl pyrophosphate

Isopentenyl pyrophosphate

$\downarrow$ $\searrow$ PPi

Geranyl pyrophosphate

Isopentenyl Pyrophosphate

$\downarrow$ $\searrow$ PPi

Farnesyl Pyrophosphate

Farnesyl pyrophosphate

$\downarrow$ $\searrow$ PPi

Presqualene

NADPH+H

$\downarrow$ NADP+PPi

Squalnene

$\downarrow$ $1/2 O_2$

Lanosterol

$\longrightarrow$ CH_3

$\longrightarrow$ 2CH_3

Cholesterol

Lipotropic agents provide methyl group for the biosynthesis of carnitine which promotes the oxidation of fatty acids.

Atherosclerosis

Deposition of lipids occur in the layers of arteries and aorta.

Gaucher's disease

Due to lack of cerebrosidase, deposition of cerebrosides occurs in liver, spleen and brain. This leads to enlargement of liver and spleen and mental deficiency.

Niemann-Pick disease

This occurs due to deficiency of sphingomyelinase. Deposition of sphingomyelin in liver and spleen leads to splenomegaly.

Role of liver in fat metabolism

Liver is a very important site for β-oxidation of fatty acids. Liver synthesizes fatty acids. Liver synthesizes cholesterol. It is the important site for cholesterol degradation in our body. Cholesterol is converted into bile acids and excreted. Liver synthesizes phospholipids.

Fatty liver

Normally liver contian 5% fat but in fatty liver the concentration of the fat in the liver goes upto 30-40%.

Starvation, diabetes mellitus, excess intake of fat etc. produces fatty liver.

Deficiency of lipotropic factors may also cause fatty liver and cirrhosis. However, alcohol ingestion in excess quantity is the major cause of cirrhosis.

Lipotropic agents

These substance reduce the excesslipid content of the fatty liver. Important lipotropic agents are choline, betaine and methionine.

QUESTIONS

1. Describe the steps involved in the digestion of lipids in the gastrointestinal tract.
2. Which is the major pathway for the metabolism of fatty acids.?
3. How propionic acid is oxidized in the body.?
4. What is the role of carnitine in fatty acid metabolism?
5. Describe the steps involved int he biosynthesis of fatty acid.
6. Which are the major sites for fatty acid synthesis?
7. How hormones influence the fat metabolism in adipose tissue?
8. What you understand by the term ketosis?
9. In which pathological condition ketone bodies appear in urine?
10. How cholesterol is synthesized in the body?
11. What are the major sites of cholestrol synthesis?
12. What is atherosclerosis?
13. What is Gaucher's disease?
14. What do you understand by the term Niemann-Pick disease?

11

PATHOLOGY OF BLOOD AND URINE

(a) Lymphocytes andplatelets: their role in health and disease

(b) Erythrocytes : Abnormal cells and their significance in disease.

(c) Abnormal constituents of urine and their significance in diseases.

(a) Lymphocytes and platelets, their role in health and disease

Lymphocytes are morphologically classified into two types; large lymphocyte and small lymphocyte. However, functionally they are classified into T-lymphocyte (T-from thymus) and B-lymphocyte (from bura of Fabricius)

Cellular immunity is mediated through the T-lymphocytes Humoral immunity is mediated throughthe B-lymphocytes. T-lymphocytes liberates interferon and lymphotoxin which are active against viral and cancer cells.

B-lymphocytes are converted into plasma cells, which liberate antibodies (immunoglobulins) which act against harmful antigens.

AIDS (Acquired immunodeficiency syndrome)

It is caused by a virus, HLTVIII (human lymphocyte Tvirus III) which resides within the T-lymphocytes and destroys the T-lymphocytes. Thus the cellular immunity is reduced severely. The patient becomes susceptible to various fatal infections.

AIDS virus is transmitted through infected needles or blood transfusion. It is also transmitted through prostitutes and other unhealthy sexual practice.

Platelets (Thrombocytes)

Platelets are very small bodies (3 μ diameter)

They are non-nucleated.

Platelets play a vital role in blood coagulation. Whenever there is damage of blood vessels platelet aggregation takes place which seals off the vessel, provided the gap is small.

Platelets also liberate many mediators likeADP, 5HT etc. which help in clotting process. If the platelet count is below 4000/cmm, hemorrhagic developement occurs. Similarly if the count is more intravascular clotting occurs in the body.

(b) Erythrocytes abnormal cells and their significance

Erythrocyte (red blood cell) does not have a nucleus. It is circular, biconcave and is very plastic. It contains hemoglobin which carries the oxygen. Anemia is the condition where the hemoglobin % is low or the erythrocyte count is less. Anemia occurs also due to blood loss or due to deficiency of elements ($Fe++$, $Cu++$) vitamins (B_{12}, Folic acid).

Anemia due to blood loss

Peptic ulcer, menstruation, piles, hook worm infestation etc cause loss of blood which leads to anemia.

Hemolytic anemia

It occurs due to bacterial infection (hemolytic streptococci) Malarial infection, snake bite and also due to drugs like primaquin in patients who have low concentration of glucose-6-phosphate dehydrogenase.

Microcytic anemia

In microcytic anemia the size of the red blood cells are small and look pale. It occurs due to the deficiency of iron.

Macrocytic anemia

The size of the RBCs is more and this occurs due to the deficiency of folic acid or B_{12}.

Aplastic Anemia

Bone marrow depression produces aplastic anemia. X-radiation, chloramphenicol, phenylbutazone etc. cause aplastic anemia.

Pernicious anemia occus due to the deficiency of intrinsic factor.

Polycythemia : A relative or absolute increase in the number of circulating red blood cells.

Hemorrhagic disorder like hemophilia can also cause anemia.

Agranulocytosis : A reduction in the number of neutrophils in the blood.

Leukemia : Neoplastic disorders of the blood forming tissue, primarily those of the leukocytic series.

(c) Abnormal Constituents of Urine and Their significance in disease.

Abnormal constituents appear in the urine sample whenever there is pathological condition of the body. The following table shows the abnormal constituents and related disorders.

Abnormal Constituent	Diseases
Albumin	Albumin is present in urine whenever there is nephritis (Kidney damage)
Bile pigment (Bilirubin)	In destruction of liver cells (Hepatitis) and obstructive jaundice
Glucose	In diabetes mellitus, endocrine disorder
Ketonebodies (Acetone, acetoacetic acid, β-hydroxy butyric acid)	In diabetes mellitus, Starvation

QUESTIONS

1. Define the term anemia.
2. What is microcytic anemia?
3. What is meant by macrocytic anemia?
4. What do you under stand by the term hemolytic anemia?
5. What is aplastic anemia?
6. What is leukemia?
7. What is meant by polycythemia?
8. Which lymphocytes liberate interferon and lymphtoxins?
9. Which lymphocytes produce antibodies?
10. What is AIDS?
11. What are the major functions of platelets?
12. In which pathological condition protein appears in the Urine?
13. How do you find out the diabetes mellitus by analysing Urine sample?
14. In which disease bile salts and bile pigments appear in urine?

SECTION — I

DETECTION AND IDENTIFICATION OF PROTEINS, AMINOACIDS, CARBOHYDRATES AND LIPIDS

Expt. 1.   Qualitative tests for proteins and aminoacids.

Expt. 2.   Qualitativetests for carbohydrates.

Expt. 3.   Qualitative tests for lipids.

EXPERIMENT — 1

QUALITATIVE TESTS FOR PROTEINS AND AMINOACIDS.

Proteins are compounds consisting of aminoacids. Proteins exhibit colloidal propertiesand therefore do not diffuse through an intact animal membrane. Hydrolysis, with acids or alkalis, breaks the protein into constituent amino acids.

Precipitation of protein by heavy metals

When solutions of salts of heavy metals are added to protein solutions a precipitate is formed. Prepare a 5% solution of egg albumin and perform the following tests.

1. To 3 ml of the egg albumin solution add mercuric chloride solution (Saturated solution), drop by drop. At first a white turbidity is produced which becomes thick and and finally granular. The precipitate dissolves after the addition of saturated solution of sodium chloride.
2. To 3 ml of the protein solution add ferric cholride (0.5%) drop by drop. On addtion of the first drop turbidity appears. Add another drop, the turbidity may increase, depending upon the concentration of the protein solution. On addition of excess ferric chloride the precipitate redissolves.
3. To 3 ml of the solution add lead acetate (2%) solution. White precipitate is formed.
4. The proteins can also be precipitated by dilute solutions of silvernitrate, bariumchloride and copper sulphate.

Precipitation of proteins by alkaloid reagents

5. To 3 ml of the protein solution add few drops of sulphosalicylic acid (20%) A white precipitate is formed.
6. To 3 ml of the solution add Esbach's reagent (consists of 1 g picric acid and 2 g of citric acid in 100 ml of water) A yellowish precipitate is formed.

7. To 3 ml of the solution add 5 drops fresh tannic acid solution (5%). A brownish precipitate is formed.

Precipitation of proteins by other reagents

Phosphotungstic acid, trichloracetic acid and phosphomolybdic acid also precipitate proteins from their solution.

To 2 ml of absolute alcohol add protein solution drop by drop. A white precipitate is formed. The precipitate does not dissolve in water due to change caused by alcohol.

Nitric acid (Heller's) test

To 3 ml of concentrated nitric acid ina test tube, add carefully, about 3 ml. of a protein solution so as to from an upper layer. Mix gently by rotating between palms. A white ring is formed at the junction of the two fluids.

Acetic acid potassium ferrocyanide test

To 3 ml of the protein solution add 3 drops of glacial acetic acid followed by 3 drops of potassium ferrocyanide. A white precipitate is obtanied.

COLOUR REACTION OF PROTEIN

1. Biuret test

To 2-3 ml of protein solution in a test tube add an equal volume of 10% sodium hydroxide solution. Mix thoroughly and add 0.5% copper sulphate solution drop by drop until a purplish-violet colour is produced (Blue precipitate of copper hydroxide is formed if excess copper sulphate is added)

Biuret reaction is due to the peptide linkage O=C-N-H or due to two carbamyl groups ($CONH_2$). Hence, it is positive with all proteins.

$$CONH_2$$
$$|$$
$$NH$$
$$|$$
$$CONH_2$$

Biuret

2. Xantho-proteic reaction

To 2-3 ml of protein solution in a test tube add 1 ml. of conc nitric acid. A white precipitate forms, and upon heating turns yellow

.and finally dissolves imparting to the solution a yellow colour. Cool the test tube and carefully add enough strong sodium hydroxide or ammonium hydroxide, to make it alkaline. The yellow colour deepens and changes to orange.

Peptones do not form precipitate with nitric acid but their solutions turn yellow and then orange when made alkaline.

The precipitate is due to the formation of metaproteins insoluble in nitric acid. The yellow colour is due to the formation of nitro-compounds from protein molecule containing benzene ring.

In alkaline medium these nitro-compounds ionise freely and produce deep yellow or orange colour. Aminoacids which give this colour reaction are Phenylalanine, tyrosine and Tryptophan. [Phenol (0.1%) will also give this type of colour change in the place of protein]

3. Glyoxylic acid reaction for tryptophan (Hopkins-Cole)

Place 2-3 ml of egg albumin solution and an equal volume of glyoxylic acid in a test tube and mix thoroughly. Incline the tube and add 5-6 ml of conc sulphuric acid to flow slowly down the side of the tube, to form a sharp layer of acid beneath protein mixture. A reddish violet colour forms at the zone of contact of two fluids. If the colour does not appear for a few minutes, give slight vibration for mixing of liquids at the interface (Solution should not be stirred, because by stirring, the precipitate of protein dissolves and violet colour spreads through out the solution). This colour is due to the presence of tryptophan group.

4. Ninhydrin reaction

To 5 ml of dilute protein solution (pH between 5 and 7) add 0.5 ml of a 0.1% solution of ninhydrin. Heat to boiling for one or two minutes and allow to cool. A blue colour appears.

This test is given by all aminoacids except proline and hydroxyproline. Proline and hydroxyproline react with ninhydrin and give yellow colour.

5. Millon's reaction

To 5 ml of protein solution add 3-4 drops of Millon's reagent and mix. Heat to boiling point over a small flame. Proteins like egg albumin. gives white precipitate which gradually turns red on heating. Proteoses and peptones give red colour. If no colour develops, add 2-3 more drops of Millon's reagentand heat again. However, large quantity of Millon's reagent givesyellow colour which is not a positive reaction. This reaction is due to the presence of the hydroxyphenyl group in protein molecule e.g. Tyrosine.

6. Millon-Nasse reaction

To 5 ml of dilute solutionof protein in a test tube add 1 ml of 15% solution of mercuric sulphate in 6 N sulphuric acid.

Place the tube in a boiling water bath for 10 minutes. Cool the contents in water for 5 to 10 minutes and add 1 ml of 1% sodium nitrite. A deep red colour indicates the presence of tyrosine.

7. The Nitroprusside test (For cysteine, cystine and methionine)

Thiol groups react with sodium nitroprusside in the presence of excess ammonia to give a red colour.

Mix 0.5 ml of a fresh solution of sodium nitroprusside with2 ml of test solution and 0.5 ml of ammonium hydroxide.

8. Sakaguchi test for arginine

Take 2-3 ml of protein solution in a test tube. Add 2 drops of α-naphthol solution(Molisch's reagent) and 1 ml of sodium hydroxide (40% solution). Mix and add 2 drops of bromine water or sodium hypobromite. A red colour indicates the presence of arginine in the protein.

9. Formaldehyde Sulphuric Acid Test

Take a little tyrosine in a test tube. Add 3 ml of Morner's reagent. (Consists of 1 ml formalin, 45 ml distilled water and 55 ml of conc Sulphuric acid).Heat gently to the boiling point. A green colour appears.

Folins Test

To 2 ml of the test solution add an equal volume of phenol reagent (Folin-Ciocalteu) and 3-10 ml of saturated solution of sodium carbonate. A blue colour is given by tyrosine.

EXPERIMENT — 2

QUALITATIVE ANALYSIS OF CARBOHYDRATES

The carbohydrates can be conveniently divided into following three groups :
1. Monosaccharides or simple sugars
2. Disaccharides
3. Polysaccharides

1. Monosaccharides

Monosaccharides are generally crystalline compounds, very soluble in water. They are the simplest carbohydrates which cannot be further broken down into smaller carbohydrates.

They are insoluble in most of the organic solvents. They are optically active.

Important sugars belonging to this group are *glucose* and *fructose*

2. Disaccharides

Disaccharides are condensation products of two monosaccharide molecules with the elimination of water. The monosac-charide molecule may be similar or disimilar.

e.g.   Maltose on hydrolysis yields two molecules of glucose Lactose on hydrolysis yields glucose+galactose. Sucrose on hydrolysis yields glucose+fructose

3. Polysaccharides

Polysaccharides are formed by condensation of a large number of monosaccharide molecules e.g. Starch, dextrin, glycogen and Inulin.

TEST FOR CARBOHYDRATES

A 1% solution is prepared to carry out the tests.

1. MOLISCH'S TEST

Reagents required

> (i) Molisch's reagent : This is prepared by dissolving 5 gm of α-naphthol in 100 ml of ethanol.
> (ii) Conc sulphuric acid.

Principle : Concentrated sulphuric acid hydrolyses glycosidic bonds of carbohydrate to give monosaccharides. The monosaccharides are then dehydrated by the acid to form furfural and it derivatives. These compounds combine with sulphonated β-naphthol to give a purple complex.

Procedure : Take 2 ml of the test solution in a test tube. Add 2 drops of Molisch's reagent. Mix. carefully pour about 1 ml of concsulphuric acid along the side of the test tube, so as to form a layer below the mixture. A red-violet ring appears which indicates the presence of carbohydrates.

2. IODINE TEST

Reagent required

Iodine solution : 0.005 normal iodine in 3% potassium iodide solution.

Principle : Acidify the test solution with dilute hydrochloric acid, then, add two drops of iodine solution and compare the colour with that of water and iodine.

> Starch gives blue colour.
>
> Glycogen gives red colour
>
> Sugars do not give change in colour.

3. BARFOED'S TEST

Reagent required : Barfoed's reagent. It consists of 13.3 gm of copper acetate in about 200 ml of water and 1.8 ml of glacial acetic acid.

Principle : Barfoed's reagent is weakly acidic and is only reduced by monosaccharides. A precipitate of cuprous oxide is obtained. Prolonged boiling may hydrolyse disaccharides to give a false positive reaction.

Procedure : Add 1 ml of test solution to 2 ml of Barfoed's reagent, boil for 1 minute in a water bath. Observe the colour change after every minute. If the precipitate is brick red with in 5-7 minutes, then the compound is a monosaccharide and if it becomes brick red after 7 minute, it is a disaccharide.

4. BIAL'S TEST

Reagent required

Bial's reagent : It consists of 1.5 gm of orcinol in 500 ml of Conc hydrochloric acid and 20 drops of a 10% solution of ferric chloride.

Principle : When pentose sugars are heated with concentrated hydrochloric acid furfural is formed which condenses with orcinol in the presence of ferric ions to give a green colour.

Procedure : Add 2 ml of test solution to 5 ml of Bial's orcinol solution and heat in a boiling water bath for a few minutes. A green colour indicates the presence of pentoses.

5. BENZIDINE TEST

To 0.5 ml of benzidine solution add a drop of unknown sample. Heat to boiling for a long time. Cool immediately in cold water. Violet colour indicates the presence of pentoses.

6. SELIWANOFF'S TEST

Reagent required : Seliwanoff's reagent. It consists of 0.05% resorcinol in 3N hydrochloric acid.

Principle : To 1 ml of the test solution add 5 ml of freshly prepared seliwanoff's reagent and warm in a boiling water bath for 1 mimute. Cherry red colour indicates the presence of ketose.

7. BENEDICT'S TEST

Reagent required : Benedict's reagent. It consists of copper sulphate 17.3 gm, sodium citrate 173 gm, Sodium carbonate

100 gm and distilled water to make up the volume upto 1000 ml. Sodium citrate and sodium carbonate are dissolved in about 750 ml of distilled water by heating. Copper sulphate is separately dissolved in 100 ml of water, and is then added to the solution of sodium citrate and sodium carbonate with continuous stirring. Finally the volume is made upto 1000 ml with distilled water.

Principle : Fehling's solution is modified to produce a single solution which is more stable.

Procedure : Take 5 ml of Benedict's reagent in a test tube. Add 8 drops of the test solution. Mix and place in a boiling water bath for 5 minutes. A green or yellow or orange-red colour indicates the presence of reducing sugars.

8. FORMATION OF OSAZONE

Reagents required

    (i) Phenylhydrazine hydrochloride

    (ii) Sodium acetate

    (iii) Glacial acetic acid

Principle : This is a test for reducing sugars. When a solution of a reducing sugar is heated with phenyhydrazine, yellow crystalline compounds called osazones are formed. Each individual sugar will give rise to an osazone of a definite crystalline form which is typical for that sugar.

Procedure

Prepare solutions of sugars as given below :

    (i) Glucose 0.5%

    (ii) Fructose 0.5%

    (iii) Lactose 2%

    (iv) Maltose 2%

    (v) Sucrose 2%

    Carry out the test with each of the solution as described below.

    To 5 ml of sugar solution in a test tube add 10 drops of glacial acetic acid. Then add a knife point of Phenylhydrazine hydrochloride and twice the amount of sodium acetate crystals. Mix well and warm a little to dissolve the solids. Filter the solution in another test tube and keep the filtrate in a boiling water bath. After 20 minutes remove the tube and examine.

Yellow crystals of glucosazone will appear in the tubes containing glucose and fructose with in 5 minute since glucosazone is insoluble even at high temperature.

Fructose behaves like glucose yielding glucosazone.Tubes containing lactose and maltose show yellow colour but no precipitate, where as sucrose solution remains unchanged.

After 20 minutes of boiling in the water bath remove the tubes and allow them to cool in the air. Osazones of maltose and lactose separate out on cooling. They are soluble in hot solution.

Sucrose does not form any osazone.

Examine the osazone crystals under a microscope.Glucosazone crystals are greenish yellow, needle shaped and are arranged in fan shape.

Lactosazone crystals are thin small needles and appear like a ball of prickles Maltosazone crystals are plate like and give an appearance like sunflower.

9. AMINOGUANIDINE REACTION

Take 0.5 ml of concentrated sulphuric acid in a test tube. Add 0.2 ml of 2.5% aqueous aminoguanidine sulphate solution without mixing. Add 0.2 ml of the test solution and mix well. A bright-reddish purple colour indicates the presence of ketohexose like fructose.

10. FERMENTATION TEST

Materials required

    (a) Fermentation tubes

    (b) Phosphate buffer (0.1 m pH 6.6)

    (c) Baker's yeast (prepare 20% suspension in buffer)

    (d) Incubator at 37°C.

Principle

Yeast ferments some carbohydrates to give alcohol and Co_2.

Prodedure

Mix equal volumeof test solution (1%) and yeast suspension and place in a fermentation tube. Incubate the tube at 37°C for 1 hr. Evolution of Co_2 indicates the presence of glucose.

11. TESTS FOR SUCROSE

Reagents required

1. Sucrose solution (1%)
2. Conc hydrochloric acid
3. Sodium hydroxide (5N)
4. Benedicts reagent
5. Seliwanoffs reagent.

Principle

Sucrose is a non-reducing disaccharide. It does not reduce alkaline copper solutions. It does not form an osazone. Sucrose is there fore hydrolysed in acid solution to glucose and fructose.

Procedure

Add 5 drops of conchydrochloricacidto 5 ml of the sucrose solution, heat for5 minute on a boiling water bath cool and add Sodium hydroxide to give slight alkalinity. Then perform Benedicts test and Seliwanoffs test.

12. ANTHRONE REACTION

Reagent required : Anthrone solution(0.2%in Conc H_2So_4)

Principle : Concentrated sulphuricacid hydrolyses glycosidic bonds to give the monosaccharides which are then dehydrated to furfural and its derivatives. The furfural reacts with anthrone to give a blue-green colour.

Procedure : Take 2 ml of the anthrone reagent in a test tube. Add 5 drops of the test solution. Mix will and observe the colour change.

EXPERIMENT — 3

QUALITATIVE TESTS FOR LIPIDS

Lipids are naturally occuring compounds that are saponifiable esters of long chain fatty acids. Lipids are insoluble in water but soluble in organic solvents such as acetone, alcohol, chloroform, benzene and ether.

1. THE SOLUBILITY OF LIPIDS

Reagents required

- (a) Fatty acids (Butyric, stearic acids)
- (b) Oils (olive oil, cod liver oil)
- (c) Solvents(Acetone, alcohol, chloroform)

Procedure

- (i) Examine the solubility of the lipids in water and in organic solvents and observe the difference in the solubility.
- (ii) Place a drop of the above mentioned oil in ether on a filter paper and leave to dry. Observe the formation of a clear grease spot.

2. SOAP FORMATION

Heat a little stearic acid with dilute alkali and observe the appearance of a soapy solution.

Testfor free fatty acid

Take 1 ml of phenolphthalein in a test tube and add carefully dilute alkali until a permanent pink colour is produced. Add this drop by drop to a solution of the test compond in ether. Discolouration of the pink colour indicates the presence of free fatty acid.

Test for unsaturation; Reagents required : olive oil, corn oil, Bromine water

Principle

Bromine readily add across the double bonds and the dicolourization of a solution of bromine by a lipid indicate the presence of double bonds.

Procedure

Slowly add bromine water to the test solution drop by drop, mixing after each addition. Bromine watargets decolourized if double bonds are present.

CHEMICAL TESTS FOR CHOLESTEROL

The Liebermann-Burchard reaction

Reagents required :

Cholesterol
Chloroform
Aceticanhydride
Sulphuric acid

Principle

Acetic anhydride reacts with cholesterol in a chloroform solution to give a characterstic green colour. Esterification of the hydroxyl group at the third position as well as other rearrangements in the molecule is responsible for the formation of chromophore.

Procedure

Take 1 ml of cholesterol solution (10 mg in 1 ml chloroform) in a test tube. Add 1 ml of aceticanhydride followed by 2 ml of conc. sulphuric acid, green colour appears.

Salkowski test

Take 1 ml of cholesterol solution in a test tube and carefully add conc sulphuric acid down the side of the tube to form two layers. The chloroform layer exhibits a red to blue colour. Whereas the acid layers shows green fluorescence.

FORMALDEHYDE TEST

Reagents required

> Cholesterol solution (10 mg/ml in chloroform)
>
> Formaldehyde (40% solution)
>
> Sulphuric acid
>
> Acetic anhydride

Principle

When formaldehyde-sulphuric acid (1 in 50) is added to a solution of cholesterol in chloroform, a red colour is formed in the chloroform layer. When acetic anhydride is added to the aqueous layer, blue colour is formed.

Procedure

Take 1 ml of cholesterol solution (10 mg/ml in chloroform) in a test tube. Add 2 ml of a solution of formaldehyde in sulphuricacid (1 in 50). A red colour is formed. Separate the aqueous layer and add 2 drops of acetic anhydride. A blue colour appears.

SECTION — II

ANALYSIS OF NORMAL AND ABNORMAL CONSTITUENTS

The majority of biochemical tests carried out in clinical laboratory is on blood, Serum and Plasma. Venous blood is always used.

Whole blood is used for the estimation of blood sugar, urea etc.

Separation of Plasma

Blood is collected in a centrifuge tube containing anticoagulant, and centrifuged. A clear straw or yellow fluid separates. This is plasma•Sodium fluoride 10 mg/ml of blood can be used as an anticoagulant.

Serum : Blood is collected in a test tube (or small bottle) with out anticoagulant. Allowed to stand for about 30 minutes to form a clot. The serum is separated from the clot by centrifugation.

EXPERIMENT — 4

ESTIMATION OF BLOOD GLUCOSE (Asatoor and King)

Principle : Protein free filtrate is heated with alkalinecopper sulphate, in a test tube. Alkaline copper sulphate is reduced byglucose to form cuprous oxide (Cu_2O). It is treated with phosphomolybdic acid to develop a blue colour. The blue colour is developed due to the reduction of the phosphomolybdic acid (Molybedenum blue). It is compared with a colour developed by a standard glucose solution.

Reagents required

1. Sodium tungstate 10% solution.

2. Reagents A : It consists of the following ingredients.
   Sodium sulphate 30 g
   Copper sulphate 6 g
   Distilled water to 1000 ml

3. Reagent B : It consists of
   Sodium potassium tartrate 12 g
   Sodium carbonate 20 g
   Sodium bicarbonate 25 g
   Potassium oxalate 18 g
   Distilled water to 1000 ml

4. Phosphomolybidic acid reagent

   Dissolve 35 g of molybidic acid and 5 g of sodium tungstate in 200 ml of distilled water and 200 ml of 10% sodium hydroxide and boil for 40 minutes to remove the ammonia. Cool and dilute the solution to 350 ml with distilled water. Add 125 ml of orthophosphoric acid. Make up the volume to 500 ml with distilled water.

Procedure

Add 0.1 ml of blood into 3.8 ml of reagent A in a test tubeand mix it.Then add 0.1 ml of 10% sodium tungstate. Mix itwell and centrifuge. To 1 ml of the supernatent liquid add 1 ml of reagent B. Plug the test tube with cotton wool and heat it on a boiling water bath for 10 minutes. Cool and add 3 ml of phosphomolybidic acid reagent and 3 ml of distilled water. Mix well and keep it for 5 minutes. Read the optical density at 680 mμ using a red filter.

Preparationof Standard

Take 1 ml of standard glucose 25 μg/ml (Prepared in Reagent A) in a test tube. Add 1 ml of reagent B. Plug the test tube with Cotton wool and heat it on a boiling water bath for 10 minutes. Cool and add 3 ml of phosphomolybidic acid reagent and 3 ml of distilled water. Mix well andkeep it for 5 minutes. Read the optical density at 680 mμ.

Preparation of Blank

Take 1 ml of reagent A in a test tube and proceed in the same way as that for the standard mentioned above.

$$\text{Mg of glucose in 100 ml of blood} = \frac{\text{Optical density of test}}{\text{Optical density of std}} \times 100$$

$$= \frac{\text{Optical density of test-optical density of blank}}{\text{Optical density of std-optical density of blank}} \times 100$$

Interpretation

Fasting blood sugar level ranges from 80-120 mgs/100ml.

The level increases in diabetes mellitus, hyperthyroidism, emotional states like fear, anger and anxiety.

Decrease in blood glucose level is observed in tumors of pancreas.

Hypoglycemia occurs in overdosage of insulin.

O-TOLUIDINE METHOD

Principle

Glucose reactswith O-toluidine in glacial acetic acid at 100°C to form a blue-green coloured compound (N-glucosylamine) which is measured colorimetrically.

Reagents required

(i) **Ortho-Toluidine Reagent :** To 5 g of thiourea add 90 ml of ortho-toluidine and dilute to 1 liter with glacial acetic acid store in a brown bottle. The reagent is stable for a year at 4-8°C.

(ii) Trichloracetic acid 10% in water.

(iii) Glucose standard 1 mg/ml.

Boil about 120 ml of distilled water. Add 2-3 spatula of benzoic acid. Mix. cool and filter. Transfer 100 mgs of glucose to 100 ml flask. Add the above solution upto 100 ml mark Mix thoroughly.

Procedure

Blank : To 1.4 ml water add 0.6 ml of 10% trichloracetic acid. Mix well.Transfer 1 ml to a test tube labeled B.

Test : To 1.2 ml of water add 0.2 ml blood and mix. Add 0.6 ml 10% trichloracetic acid. Mix well,wait for 5 minutes. Centrifuge for 10 minutes. Transfer 1 ml clear supernatant liquid to a test tube labeled T.

Standard : To 1.2 ml water add 0.2 ml glucose standard solution followed by 0.6 ml 10% trichloracetic acid. Mix well transfer 1 ml to a test tube labeled S.

To all the three tubes add 5 ml each of ortho-toluidine reagent and mix. Place them in boiling water bath for 10 minutes cool read optical densites of B, S and T using red filter.

$$\text{Mgs of glucose per 100 ml} = \frac{\text{O.D of Test-0.D of Blank}}{\text{O.D of S-O.D of B}} \times 100$$

Precautions

1. O-toluidine is highly corrosive. Use gloves while handling this chemical.

2. Use automatic dispensers for O-toluidine reagent.

Glucose Tolerance Test (GTT)

Glucose tolerance Test is done to find out the ability of the body to utilise an additional load of glucose given orally. The glucose given is utilised faster in normal persons than in diabetic patients. There is delay in removal of glucose in diabetics. This is due to deficiency of insulin.

A comparison of the tolerance curve of a normal person with that of diabetic patient gives an idea of the severity of diabetes.

Patient Preparation

The patient should be asked to take usual diet for at least three days precedding the test. On the day prior to the performance of test instruct the patient not to take any thing, except water, after 8 O' clock in the night. Ask the patient to come to the laboratoty the next morning at 8 O' clock. This means, the patient should be asked to observe fast for 12 hrs before test.

Method of conducting test

Collect fasting blood and urine samples. Dissolve 50 g of glucose in 300 ml of water, ask the patient to drink the glucose solution. Note the time. Collect four more samples of blood and urine after every half an hour. After the ingestion of glucose (upto 2 hrs). analyse all the samples for their glucose content. Perform Benedict's qualitative test on the urine sample.

Construct a curve on a graph sheet by plotting concentration of blood sugar (mg%) on Y-axis and time on x-axis.

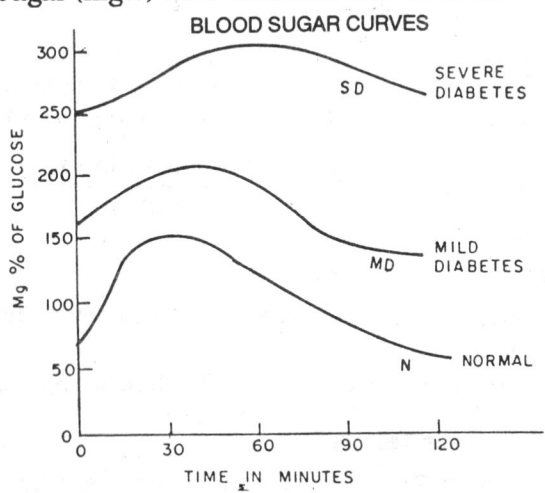

BLOOD SUGAR CURVES

Interpretation

In a normalperson (Curve N) the fasting blood sugar level is between 80-120 mg%. It does not rise above 160 mg%. Sugar is absent in urine sample. In mild diabetes mellitus (curve MD) the fasting blood glucose level is slightly higher than 120 mg%. It rises above 160 mg% at 60 minutes and the level comes down below 160 mg% at the end of 120 minutes. At least one of the urine samples show positive reaction with Benedict's reagent. In Severe diabetis mellitus curve (SD), the fasting blood sugar level is much higher (More than 200 mg%). The glucose level crosses 300 mgs/100ml in 60 minutes. The fall in glucose is very small due to lack of insulin. All the urine samples show positive reaction with Benedicts reagent.

EXPERIMENT — 5

ESTIMATION OF UREA IN BLOOD (Nesslerisation Method)

Principle

The Urease enzyme hydrolyses Urea to ammonium carbonate which on treatment with Nessler"s reagent produces yellowish orange colour. The absorbance of the colour produced is measured colourimetrically using green filter at 540 nm.

$$\underset{\text{Urea}}{\overset{H_2N}{\underset{H_2N}{\diagup}}\hspace{-0.5em}C=0} \xrightarrow{\text{Urease}} 2NH_3 + Co_2 \xrightarrow{+H_2O} (NH_4)_2\,Co_3$$

Reagents required

1. Sodium tungstate 10% solution in water.
2. Sulphuric acid 0.667 N
3. Nessler's reagent.

   Add 50 g mercuric iodide, 35 g potassium iodide and 200 ml distilled water into a 500 ml volumetric flask mix to dissolve.

   In a beaker dissolve 50 g sodium hydroxide in 250 ml of water. Add this solution to volumetric flask with stirring and make upto 500 ml with water. Use the clear supernatant.

4. Urease suspension

   Grind 1 g horse gram powder with 10 ml water and 500 mgs of potassium chloride. Use supernatant. Keep in refrigerator.

5. Standard Urea solution

Dissolve 60 mgs Urea in water and make upto 100 ml. Store in refrigerator. Prepare fresh every week.

Procedure

Take two centrifuge tubes and label them as T and S.

Add 0.5 ml blood and 3 ml water into the centrifuge tube labeled as T. Add 0.5 ml standard and 3 ml water into S. Incubate at 55°C for 5 minutes. Pipet 0.5 ml each of urease suspension to T and S. Note the time. Incubate at 50°C for 5 minutes.

Stop enzyme reaction by adding 0.5 ml of 0.667 N Sulphuric acid to T and S. Mix, allow to stand for 3 minutes. Add 0.5 ml of 10% sodium tungstate to T and S. Mix. centrifuge at 2000 r.p.m. for 5 minutes. Take 3 test tubes and label them as B, S and T Add 7 ml of water into B. Pipet 2 ml of the supernatant from centrifuge tube S into S tube and add 5 ml of water. Mix Prepare test in the same way.

Add 1 ml Nessler's reagent to B and read the optical density using green filter or 540 nm in a colorimeter.

Add 1 ml Nesslers reagent to T and take reading.

Add 1 ml Nesslers reagent to S and take reading.

Calculations

$$\text{Mgs urea per 100 ml} = \frac{\text{Reading of T} - \text{Reading of B}}{\text{Reading of S} - \text{Reading of B}} \times 0.12 \times \frac{100}{0.2}$$

$$= \frac{\text{O.D of T} - \text{O.D of B}}{\text{O.D of S} - \text{O.D of B}} \times 60$$

Precautions

1. Do no mix after adding Nesslers reagent. It may form turbidity.
2. To avoid turbidity formation add one drop of saturated sodium potassium tartrate solution.
3. Ammonium oxalate should not be used as an anticoagulant.

Diacetyl monoxime method

Principle : Urea reacts with diacetyl monoxime under strong acidic conditions in presence of ferric ions and thiosemicarbazide to give pink coloured complex.

Reagents required

1. Diacetyl monoxime Dissove 1.56 g diacetyl monoxime in 250 ml water.

2. **Ferric chloride :** Dissolve 324 mgs of ferric chloride in 10 ml of 56% orthophosphoric acid. Preserve in brown bottle.

3. **Thiosemicarbazide :** Dissolve 41 mgs of thiosemicarbazide in 250 ml of water.

4. **Sulphuric acid 20% :** Add 200 ml of conc sulphuric acid to 800 ml of water in a beaker with stirring and cooling.

5. **Acid reagent :** To 1000 ml of 20% sulphuric acid add 1 ml of ferric chloride reagent.

6. Trichloracetic acid 10%

7. **Preservative diluents for standard :** Heat about 250 ml water. Add 40 mgs of phenylmercuric acetate. Mix well to dissolve the substance. Transfer to 1 liter flask. Add 0.3 ml conc sulphuric acid and makeup the volume to 1000 ml.

8. Standard Urea 0.1 mg/ml (100 µg/ml). Dissolve 10 mg of urea in 100 mlof preservative diluent.

Procedure

Test : Take 3.4 ml of distilled water in a test tube and add 0.1 mlof blood and mix. Add 1.5 ml of 10% trichloracetic acid. mix well and allow it to stand for 5 minutes. Centrifuge at 2000 r.p.m. for 5 minutes. Take 1 ml of the supernatant and pipet into a test tube labeled asT.

Standard : Take 1 ml of the standard urea in a test tube labeled as S.

Blank : Pipet 1 ml of water in a test tube labeled as B.

Add 1 ml of each of diacetylmonoxime to B,S, and T.

Add 1 mlof thiosemicarbazide, followed by 3 ml of acid reagent to B, S and T. and mix well. Keep the three tubes (B, S and T) in a boiling water bath for exactly 15 mimutes cool. Read optical density using green filter or at 540 nm setting the readingto zero with water.

$$\text{Mgs of urea in 100 ml blood} = \frac{\text{O.D of T} - \text{O.D of B}}{\text{O.D of S} - \text{O.D of B}} \times 0.01 \times \frac{100}{0.2}$$

Significances of Urea Estimation

Normal blood urea ranges form 15-45 mgs per100 ml. The level is influenced by the proteins in the diet. Urea level is decreased on low protein die. Urea level is higher on high protein diet.

Increases are seen in :

    (i) Acute and chronic nephritis and renal failure.

    (ii) Renal tuberculosis

    (iii) Renal cancer

    (iv) Hemoconcentration due to severe vomiting and diarrhoea and in burns.

    (v) Fever.

EXPERIMENT — 6 & 7

ESTIMATION OF CREATININE IN BLOOD

Principle

By Jaffe's Reaction

Creatinine gives an amber colour on reaction with picric acid in the presence of strong alkali. the amber colour is due to the formation of creatinine picrate.

REAGENTS REQUIRED

1. Standard Creatinine Solution (Stock)

Prepare a stock standard Creatinine by dissolving 100 mgs of pure dry creatinine in N/10 hydrcholoric acid and dilute to 100 ml with N/10 hydrochloric acid. This solution is very stable and contains 1 mg of creatinine per ml.

2. Creatinine Working Standard (50 µg/ml)

1. Take 5 ml of the stock solution in a volumetric flask. Add 10 ml of N/10 hydrochloric acid and make upto 100 ml with distilled water.
2. Picric acid 1% solutionprepared in distilled water.
4. Sodium hydroxide-10% solutionprepared in distilled water.
5. Sodium tungstate-10% solution prepared in distilled water.
6. Sulphuric acid 2/3 N.

Procedure

Take 7 ml of water in a test tube. Add 1 ml of serum and 1 ml of 10% sodium tungstate. mix. Add 1 ml of 2/3 N sulphuric acid with constant shaking. Allow it to stand for a few minutes, centrifuge and filter. Take 5 ml of the filtrate into a tube labeled as T. Take 0.2 ml of standard creatinine (50 µg/ml) in a test tube labeled as S. and make up the volume upto 5 ml with distilledwater. Take5 ml of water in a tube labeled as B. Add 2 ml of 1% picricacid followed by 0.15 ml of 10% sodium hydroxide solution. Mix gently and allow to stand for 15 minutes. Transfer a portion of the blank and adjust the colorimeter to zero O.Dat 520 nm. Then take the reading for standard and unknown sample.

$$\text{Serum Creatinine (mg/100ml)} = \frac{\text{O.D of Test}}{\text{O.D of Std}} \times \frac{0.01}{0.5} \times 100$$

$$= \frac{\text{O.D of Test}}{\text{O.D of Std}} \times 2$$

Significances

Normal levelof cretinine in serum is 0.6-1.5 mg/100ml.

Serum creatinine increases in renal failure.

Estimation of Urine Creatinine

Urine creatinine is estimated in the same way as serum creatinine.There is no need for precipitation of protein with sodium tungstate. Urine should be diluted (1in 100) before the estimation.

Procedure for the Estimation of Creatinine in Urine

Take different volumes of creatinine working standard solution (50 µg/ml) like 0.1 ml, 0.2 ml, 0.4 ml, 0.8 ml and 2 ml in 5 test tubesand in the 6th test tube take 1 ml of distilled water. Make up to volume in the other 5 test tubes upto 1 ml with distilled water, where necessary. Add 2 ml of picric acid followed by 0.15 ml of 10% sodium hydroxide solution. mix gently and allow to stand for 15 minutes and make up the volume upto 10 ml with distilled water. Transfer a portion of the blank and adjust the photometer to zero optical density at 520 mµ. Then takethe reading for standard and unknown sample. Plot a graph for standard, taking optical density Vs concentration. From the graph calculate the concentration of the test sample.

Significances of Creatinine Estimation

Creatinine is formed from creatine phosphate in the muscle and the normalexcretion of creatinine in the urine per day is 1 to 1.8 g. The excretion of creatinine gives the efficiency of renal function e.g. Excretion of creatinine is decreased in renal insufficiency and in hypothyroidisim. The creatinine, excretion is increased in hyperthyroidism, starvation, and in muscular dystrophies.

Special Note

1. Instead of test tubes volumetic flasks can be used.
2. If the time allowed for doing the practical is less, then the following calculation can be used for determining the concentration of the unknown sample.

$$\text{Conc of test per ml} = \frac{\text{0.D of Test}}{\text{0.D of Std.}} \times \text{Conc of Std per ml.}$$

ESTIMATION OF CREATINE IN URINE

Principle

Creatine when boiled with an acid is converted into its anhydride creatinine by ring closure. The creatinine already present Preformed) and that formed from the creatine are then estimated together. The preformed creatinine is estimated separately. By calculating the difference the amount of creatine is estimated.

Procedure

Pipet 0.5 ml of urine in a 250 ml flask. Add 10 ml picric acid and 150 ml of water. Boil gently for 45 minutes, Then rapidly, till the volume is reduced to 10 ml. cool the solution and proceed as for creatinine.

EXPERIMENT — 8

ESTIMATION OF BLOOD CHOLESTEROL

Principle

Blood or serum is extracted with an alcohol-acetone mixture which removes cholesterol and other lipids and precipitates protein. The organic solvent is removed by evaporation on a boiling water bath. The residue is dissolved in chloroform and colour developed by the Liebermann-Burchard reaction and compared with the standard.

Reagents required

1. Alcohol acetone mixture (1:1)
2. Chloroform (AR)
3. Acetic anhydride
4. Conc sulphuric acid
5. Standard cholesterol 0.1 mg/ml:Dissolve 10 mg of pure cholesterol in chloroform and diluted to 100 ml with chloroform.
6. Absolutely dry glassware.

Procedure

Place 10 ml of the alcohol-acetone solvent in a centrifuge tube and add 0.2 ml of serum or blood. Cork the tube and immerse the tube in a boiling water bath with shaking until the solvent begins to boil. Remove the tube and continue shaking the mixture for further 5 minutes. Cool to room temperature and centrifuge it at 1500 r.p.m. for 5 minutes Decant the supernatant fluid in a smallbeaker, andevaporate to dryness on a boiling water bath or a hot plate. Cool and disslove the residue in 6 ml of chloroform. and transfer it to a dry test tube. At the same time, label. two other test tubes, 'standard' and Blank, add 6 ml of cholesterol working standard into the standard tube. Take 6 ml of pure chloroform in the blank tube. Add 2 ml of acetic anhydride and 0.1 ml of conc sulphuric acid to all tubes and thoroughly mix. Leave the tubes in the dark at room temperature for 15 minutes and read the extinction at 680 mn. Set the photometer to zero optical density with blank.

Calculation

$$\text{Serum cholesterol (mg/100ml)} = \frac{\text{O.D of Test}}{\text{O.D of Std}} \times 0.6 \times \frac{100}{0.2}$$

$$= \frac{\text{O.D of Test}}{\text{O.D of Std.}} \times 300$$

DIRECT METHOD OF KIM AND GOLD BERG

Principle

Serum is mixed with stable Liebermann-Burchard reagent. Acetic acid in the reagent dissolves cholesterol which later, under-goes Liebermann-Burchard reaction.

REAGENT REQUIRED

1. Standard cholesterol solution

Dissolve 200 mg of cholesterol in a little quantity of glacial acetic acid in a 100 ml volumetric flask and make up the volume upto 100 ml with glacial acetic acid.

2. Stable Lieberman-Burchard reagent

Add 220 ml of ice cold acetic anhydride with 200 ml of glacial acetic acid. Then add 30 ml of ice cold conc sulphuric acid. Store the reagent in a brown bottle at 4°c.

Procedure

Take 3 test tubes and label them as blank, standard and Test.

Blank : Take 0.1 ml glacialacetic acid and 6 ml of stable Liebermann-Burchard reagent.

Standard : Take 0.1 ml of standard cholesterol solution and 6 ml of stable Liebermann-Burchard reagent.

Test : Take 0.1 ml of serum and 6 ml of stable Liebermann-Burchard reagent. Mix well a-nd incubate all tubes at 37°C for 18 minutes.Set the photometer to zero optical density with blank and read the optical density at 620 mµ.

$$\text{Serum cholesterol (mg/100 ml)} = \frac{\text{O.D of test}}{\text{O.D of Std}} \times \frac{0.2}{0.1} \times 100$$

$$= \frac{\text{O.D of test}}{\text{O.D of Std}} \times 200$$

Significances of Cholesterol estimation

The normal serum cholesterol lies within the range of 100-240mg/100ml in healthy young adults. The average serum cholesterol level is about 200 mg/100ml at 25 in men and rises slowly with age, reaching a peak figure at the age 40-50 and then declining.

A high serum cholesterol of 300 mg/100ml or more in young adults is a serious indication of coronary disease.

Serum cholesterol increases in many pathological conditions like nephrosis, lipemia, diabetes mellitus, hypothyroidisim, biliary obstruction, hepatitis and xanthomatosis. Prolonged hypercholesterolemia predisposes an individual to atherosclerosis.

Decreased serum cholesterol is found in hyperthyroidism, pernicious anemia, hepatocellular damage, wasting disease and acute infections.

EXPERIMENT — 9 & 10

ESTIMATION OF PHOSPHATASES

Phosphatases are enzymes which catalyse the splitting off of phosphoric acid from mono-phosphoric acid esters. There are two types of phosphatase present in serum, alkaline phosphatase with maximum activity at about pH 10 and acid phosphatase with maximum activity at about pH_5.

DETERMINATION OF ALKALINE PHOSPHATASE

Principle

Disodium phenylphosphate is used as a substrate and the amount of phenol released by enzymatic hydrolysis is measured colourimetrically. phenol reacts with 4-amino-phenazone (4 aminoantipyrin) to give a condensation product which is then oxidized by potassium ferricyanide to a coloured quinone.

REAGENTS REQUIRED

1. **Buffer (PH 9.90 at 37°C)** : Dissolve 3.1 g of anhydrous sodium carbonate and 1.68 g of sodium bicarbonate in water and make upto 500 ml. keep at4°C.

2. Disodium phenylphosphate (0.01 m) (Substrate):1.09 g of disodium phenyl phosphate is dissolved in 500 ml of boiled and cooled distilled water. Add 2 ml of chloroform as preservative. The substrate is stored at 4°C until required.

3. Stock standard phenol (0.1% in 0.1N HCl);keep in a brown bottle. at 4°C. It is stable for 1 month.

4. Working standard phenol 0.05 mg/ml. Dilute phenol standard to 100 ml with distilled water. Preserve with a few drops of chloroform and keep at 4°C in a brown bottle. It is stable for 1 week.

5. Sodium hydroxide 0.4 N.
6. Sodium bicarbonate 0.6 N
7. 4-amino-phenazone (4-aminoantipyrine) 0.6% in distilled water. Store in a brown bottle.
8. Potassium ferricyanide 0.4% in distilled water store in a brown bottle.

Procedure

Test : Mix 1 ml of buffer with 1 ml substrate (Disodium phenyl phosphate) in a test tube and place in a water bath at 37°C +- 0.02°C for 3 minutes. Add 0.1 ml of serum, mix gently and incubate for 15 minutes. Stop reaction by the addition of 1 ml of 0.4 N sodium hydroxide.

Control : In a test tube add 1 ml of buffer, 1 ml of substrate and 1 ml of 0.4 N NaOH followed by 0.1 ml of serum.

Standard : In a test tube mix 1 ml of buffer with 0.5 ml of Standard (0.05 mg/ml) and 0.6 ml of distilled water followed by 1 ml 0.4 NaOH.

Blank : Mix 1 ml buffer, 1.1 ml water and 1 ml 0.4 N NaOH

To each tube add 1 ml of 0.6 N Sodium bicarbonate followed by 1 ml of potassium ferricyanide solution, mixing each tube well after each addition. A reddish-brown chromophore appears at alkaline pH. Read O.D at 510 nm using green filter. Avoid exposure to strong sunlight.

The amount of phenol present in the standard tube is 25 µg.

Phenol produced in 15 minutes in the tube is

$$\frac{\text{O.D of T} - \text{O.D of Control}}{\text{O.D of Std} - \text{O.D of Blank}} \times 25 \text{ microgram}$$

∴ 100 ml of serum would liberate

$$\frac{\text{O.D of T} - \text{O.D of C}}{\text{O.D of Std} - \text{O.D of B}} \times 25 \text{ mgs of phenol}$$

Since 1 king Armstrong unit is the production of 1 mg of phenol in 15 minutes under the conditions of the test.

Serum alkaline phosphate in K.A Units/100ml.

$$= \frac{T - C}{S - B} \times 25$$

Significances

The normal range of serum alkaline phosphatase is 3-17 K A units/100 ml in adults and 17-33 KA units/100ml in children. Serum alkaline phosphatase increases in jaundice in both infective and post-hepatic obstructive jaundice. However, the rise is usually more in obstructive jaundice than in jaundice due to hepatitis.

The activity is also raised in livercancer, bone cancer, osteomalacia, rickets and hyperparathyroidism.

A decrease inserum alkaline phosphatase occurs in cretinisim, scurvy, severe anemia, and hypophosphatasia.

Estimation of Acid phosphatase

The King-Armstrong method for alkaline phosphatase was followed for acid phosphatase estimation by Gutman and Gutman, which substitute a different buffer so that the reaction could be carried out at pH 4.9.

Reagents

Same as for alkaline phosphatase except buffer.

Citric acid : Sodium citrate buffer 0.1 M pH 4.9. Dissolve21 grams of crystalline citric acid in water and add 188 ml of 1 N Sodium hydroxide and make up to 500 ml with water Adjust the pH to 4.9 by adding Normal sodium hydroxide or hydrochloric acid.

Procedure : Same as given for alkaline phosphatase except the incubation period. The incubation period is 60 minutes.

Calculation

Same as given for alkaline phosphatase

Significance

The normal range of serum acid phosphatase is 1-5 KA units/ 100 ml.

It increases in prostatic cancer.

EXPERIMENT — 11

ESTIMATION OF SERUM TOTAL AND DIRECT BILIRUBIN

Principle

Bilirubin is converted to purple-colour azo-bilirubin on treatment with diazotised sulfanilic acid.

Total bilirubin is estimated in methanolic solution.

Reagents required

1. Methanol, AR grade
2. Hydrochloric acid, 1.5% in distilled water Dilute 1.5 ml of conc hydrochloric acid to 100 ml with distilled water.
3. **Solution A :** Take 985 ml of distilled water in 1 liter flask. Add 15 ml of conc hydrochloric acid. Dissolve 1 g of sulphanilic acid in the above solution.
4. **Solution B :** Dissolve 0.5 g of sodium nitrite in water and make up the volume to 100 ml.
5. **Diazoreagent (Prepare fresh) :** Add 0.3 ml of solution B to of 10 ml of solution A and mix.
6. Standard bilirubin solution 0.1 mg/ml. Dissolve 10 mg of bilirubin in 100 ml of methanol. Store in brown bottle.

Procedure

Dilute 1 ml of serum to 20 ml with water in a conical flask and mix.

Total Bilirubin

Take two test tubes and label them as Test (Tt) and Blank (Tb).

Add 5 ml of methanol, 1 ml of 1.5% hydrochloric acid and 4 ml of diluted serum into the test tube labeled as Tb Mix well.

Add 5 ml of methanol, 1 ml of diazoreagent and 4 ml of diluted serum into the test tube labeled as Tt.mix well.

Keep both the tubes at room temperature for 30 minutes. After 30 minutes read optical density using green filter or at 540 nm.

Direct Bilirubin

Label two test tubes as Test (T_D) and Blank (D_B).

Add 5 ml of water, 1 ml of 1.5% hydrochloric acid and 4 ml of diluted serum into test tube labeled as Blank(D_B) mix well.

Add 5 ml of water, 1ml of diazoreagent and 4 ml of diluted serum into the test tube labeled as Test (T_D) mix well.

Keep both the tubes at room temperature for 30 minutes. Read optical density at 540 nm using green filter.

Take two test tubes and label them as standard (S) and Blank (S_B). Add 8.8 ml of methanol, 1 ml of diazo reagent and 0.2 ml of standard into the test tube labeled as S. mix well.

Add 8.8 ml of methanol, 1 ml of 1.5% hydrochloric acid and 0.2 ml of standard into the test tube labeled as B (S_B). Mix well.

Keep both the tubes at room temperature for 30 minutes. Read optical density at 540 nm or using green filter.

Calculation

mgs of Total Bilirubin per 100ml serum

$$= \frac{\text{0.D of } T_T - \text{0.D of } T_B}{\text{0.D of S} - \text{0.D of } S_B} \times 0.02 \times \frac{100}{0.2}$$

$$= \frac{\text{0.D of } T_T - \text{0.D of } T_B}{\text{0.D of S} - \text{0.D of } S_B} \times 10$$

mgs of Direct Bilirubin per 100 ml serum

$$= \frac{\text{0.D of } T_D - \text{0.D of } D_B}{\text{0.D of S} - \text{0.D of } S_B} \times 10$$

Significances

Direct bilirubin is water soluble conjugated bilirubin. Free bilirubin or water insoluble bilirubin (But soluble in methanol) is unconjugated bilirubin.

Normal range of serum total bilirubin is 0.2 to 0.6 mg/100 ml. Direct bilirubin in serum ranges from 0.1 to 0.4 mg/100 ml. Hyperbilirubinemia is a characteristic of Jaundice. In hemolytic jaundice and neonatal jaundice, usually unconjugated bilirubin level increases without corresponding increase in conjugated bilirubin. In viral hepatitis, toxic hepatitis and cirrhosis there is over all damage to liver cells, hence the ability of liver to form conjugated bilirubin decreases, resulting in an increase in unconjugated bilirubin in serum. In obstructive jaundice there is an increase in both conjugated and unconjugated bilirubin.

EXPERIMENT — 12

ESTIMATION OF SERUM GLUTAMATE PYRUVATE TRANSAMINASE (SGPT or Alanine Transaminase) (ALAT or ALT)

REITMAN-FRANKEL METHOD

Principle

Alanine transaminase catalyses the conversion of L-alanine to pyruvate at a temperature of 37°C.

L-alanine+ α-ketoglutaric acid → Pyruvate+glutamic acid. The pyruvate liberated is treated with dinitrophenylhydrazine to give a brown colour compound. the enzyme activity is determined using sodium pyruvate calibration standard.

REAGENTS REQUIRED

1. Phosphate buffer 0.1 M, PH 7.4

Dissolve 13.97 g of dipotassium hydrogen phosphate and 2.69 g of potassium dihydrogen phosphate in water and make upto litre with distilled water. Adjust the PH to 7.4 Store at 4°C.

2. α-Ketoglutaric acid

Dissolve 292 mgs of α-ketoglutaric acid in a little of water, adjust the pH to 7.4 with 1 N Sodium hydroxide and make up the volume to 100 ml with distilled water. Store in a refrigerator.

3. GPT substrate

Weigh 445 mgs of L-alanine. Add 5 ml of 1 N sodium hydroxide slowly with mixing, 2.5 ml of alpha-ketoglutaric a-cid and 17.5 ml of phosphate buffer, mix well. Adjust the pH to 7.4 by adding sodium hydroxide or phosphoric acid. Keep the solution in deep-freezer.

4. Pyruvate standard for calibration

Dissolve 22 mgs of sodium pyruvate in 100 ml phosphate buffer. Store in deep-freezer.

5. 2, 4-dinitrophenyl hydrazine reagent.

Dissolve 19.8 mgs of 2, 4 dinitrophenyl hydrazine in 100 ml of 1 N hydrochloric acid. Keep it in brown colour bottle.

6. Sodium hydroxide 0.4N

Dissolve 16 g of sodium hydroxide in water and dilute to 1000 ml with distilled water and store in polythene bottle.

7. Sodium hydroxide 1N

Dissolve 40 g of Sodium hydroxide in water and make up the volume to 1000 ml with distilled water.

8. Hydrochloric acid 1N

Dilute 45 ml of concentrated hydrochloric acid to 500 ml with distilled water.

Procedure

Test : Add 0.5 ml of GPT substrate into a test tube labeled as T Keep the test tube in a water bath at 37°C for 5 minutes.

Add 0.1 ml of serum and mix, keeping inside the water bath.

Incubate for exactly 30 minutes.

Add 0.5 ml of 2, 4 dinitrophenyl hydrazine solution at the end of 30 minutes.

Control : Take a test tube and mark as 'C' (Control). Add 0.5 ml GPT substrate, 0.5 ml 2, 4 dinitrophenyl hydrazine and 0.1 ml boiled serum. Mix. Keep both the tubes at room termperature for 20 minutes.

Add 5 ml of 0.4 N Sodium hydroxide to both T and C.

After 5minutes read the optical density at 505 nm or using green filter against water.

Preparation of Calibration Curve

Take six test tubes and label them as 1, 2, 3, 4, 5 and 6. Add the solutions into each tube as given below in the table.

Tube No.	Std pyruvate Solution	GPT Substrate	Water	Optical Density
1.	0	1 ml	0.2 ml	
2.	0.1 ml	0.9 ml	0.2 ml	
3.	0.2 ml	0.8 ml	0.2 ml	
4.	0.3 ml	0.7 ml	0.2 ml	
5.	0.4 ml	0.6 ml	0.2 ml	
6.	0.5 ml	0.5 ml	0.2 ml	

Add 1 ml 2, 4 dinitrophenyl hydrazine to all tubes. Allow to stand for 20 minutes at room temperatureAdd 10 ml 0.4 N sodium hydroxide, wait for 5minutes. Read optical density at505 nm or using green filter.

Draw a calibration curve by taking units on x-axis and O.D on Y-axis.

Tube No.	Optical density	GPT units (Sigma-Frankel units)
1		0
2		23
3		30
4		83
5		125

Calculate the enzyme level in units per 100 ml of the test from the graph.

Significance

Normal range of SGPT is 35 Sigma-Frankelunits (SF unit/100 ml). The level is increased in liver diseases.

EXPERIMENT — 13

ESTIMATION OF SERUM GLUTAMATE-OXALOACETATE TRANSAMINASE (SGOTor Aspartate transaminase)

REITMAN-FRANKEL METHOD

Principle

Aspartate transaminase catalyses the conversion of DL-aspartic acid to oxaloacetate at temperature of 37°C.

DL-Asparticacid + alpha-ketoglutaric acid $\longrightarrow$ oxaloacetic acid + glutamate.

The oxaloacetate formed is spontaneously converted to pyruvate which forms a brown colour with 2, 4 dinitrophenyl hydrazine.

REAGENTS REQUIRED

1. **Phosphate buffer 0.1 M PH 7.4 :** Dissolve 13.97 g of dipotassium hydrogen phosphate (K_2HPo_4) and 2.69 g of potassium dihydrogen phosphate (KH_2PO_4) in water and make upto 1 liter. Adjust the pH to 7.4 Store at 4°C.

2. **Alpha-ketoglutaric acid :** Dissolve 292 mgs of alpha ketoglutaric acid in 1000 ml of water. Adjust the pH to 7.4 with 1N Sodium hydroxide and make up the volume to 100 ml. Store in deepfreezer.

3. **GOT substrate :** Weigh 665 mgs of DL-aspartic acid or 332.5 mgs of L-aspartic acid in a volumetric flask. Add 5 ml of 1 N sodium hydroxide, 2.5 ml. of alpha-ketoglutaric acid and17.5 ml of phosphate buffer. Mix well to dissolve. Adjust the pH to 7.4 using 1 N sodium hydroxide or phosphoricacid. Keep in a freezer.

4. **Sodium pyruvate standard for calibration :** Dissolve 22 mgs of sodium pyruvate in 100 ml of phosphate buffer.
5. **2, 4-dinitrophenylhydrazine (Colour reagent) :** Dissolve 19.8 mgs of 2, 4 dinitrophenyl hydrazine in 100 ml of 1 N hydrochloric acid. Keep in a brown coloured bottle.
6. **Sodium hydroxide 1 N :** Dissolve 40 g sodium hydroxide in water and make up the volume to 1000 ml.
7. **Sodium hydroxide 0.4 N :** Dissolve 1.6 g sodium hydroxide in water and dilute to 100 ml.
8. **Hydrochloric a cid 1 N :** Dilute 9 ml of conc hydrochloric acid to 100 ml with distilled water.

Procedure

Add 0.5 ml of GOT substrate into a test tube marked as test (T). Keep in water bath at 37°C for 5 minutes. Add 0.1 ml of serum and mix, keep the tube in the water bath and incubate for 60 minutes.

Add 0.5 ml of 2.4 dinitrophenyl hydrazine after 60 minutes of incubation.

Take another test tube and mark it as Control (C) Add 0.5 ml of GOT substrate, 0.5 ml of 2, 4 dinitrophenyl hydrazine and 0.1 ml of serum and mix.

Keep both the tubes at room temperature for 20 minutes. Add 5 ml of 0.4 N Sodium hydroxide to both tubes, mix well. After 5 minutes read the optical density at 505 nm or using green filter.

Calibration of Standard

Take six tubes and number them as 1, 2, 3, 4, 5 and 6. Add the reagents into each tube as given below in the table.

Tube No.	Standard Sodium pyruvate	GOT substrate	Water
1	0	1 ml	0.2 ml
2	0.1 ml	0.9 ml	0.2 ml
3	0.2 ml	0.8 ml	0.2 ml
4	0.3 ml	0.7 ml	0.2 ml
5	0.4 ml	0.6 ml	0.2 ml
6	0.5 ml	0.5 ml	0.2 ml

Add 1 ml 2, 4 dinitrophenyl hydrazine reagent to all tubes keep them at room temperature for 20 minutes. Add 10 ml of 0.4 N sodium hydroxide to all tubes and mix. Keep the tubes for another 5 minutes. Read the optical density at 505 nm or using green filter.

Tube No.	Optical density	GOT units/100 ml
1.		0
2.		20
3.		55
4.		95
5.		148
6.		216

Draw a calibration curve by plotting units per 100 ml on x-axis and optical density on y-axis; calculate the enzyme level in units per 100 ml of test from the graph.

Note : If the SGOT levels is higher than 215 units per 100 ml repeat the test after diluting the serum with normal saline (Apply the dilution factor in the final calculation).

Significances

Normal level of this enzyme is upto 35 S F units per 100 ml. SGOT level increases in infective, toxic and viral hepatitis. SGOT is raised in myocardial infarction SGOT increases after 6 hrs of attack and reaches maximum after 12-36 hours and returns to normal after 6 days.

EXPERIMENT — 14

ESTIMATION OF SERUM CALCIUM

Principle

Calcium in the serum forms a violet coloured complex with O-cresolphthalein complexene. 8-hydroxyquineline is included in the reagent to prevent inter-ference by magnesium.

REAGENTS REQUIRED

Reagent A

Add 210 g of diethanelemine and 300 g of urea to about 900 ml of double distilled water in a beaker. Dissolve the crystals.Adjust the pH to 11.7 with acetic acid. Make up the volume to 1000 ml with double distilled water.

Reagent B

Dissolve 64 mg of O-cresolphthalein complexene, 1.68 g of 8-hydroxyquineline and 2.5 ml glacial acetic acid in 250 ml of ethanol.

Add 300 g of urea to this solution and make up the volume to 1 liter with double distilled water.

Working Reagent

Mix equal volumes of reagent A and Reagent B just before use.

Standard calcium 10 mg/ml or 5 milli Equivalent/liter
Dissolve 25 mg of dry calcium carbonate in 8 ml of N/10 hydrochloric acid and dilute to 100 ml with distilled water.

Procedure

Add 0.2 ml of serum and 1.8 ml of double distilled water in a test tube and mix. Transfer 0.5 ml of this to a test tube marked as Test (T). Add 5 ml of working reagent.

Take another test tube. Add 0.2 ml of calcium standard solution and 1.8 ml of water. Transfer 0.5 ml from this to a test tube marked as standard (S).

Add 5 ml of working reagent. Mix.

Label a 3rd test tube as blank (B) and add 0.5 ml water and 5 ml of working reagent. Mix.

Read optical densites of B, S, and T at 540 nm or using green filter.

Calculation

$$\text{mgs of calcium per 100 ml serum} = \frac{\text{O.D of T} - \text{O.D of B}}{\text{O.D of S} - \text{O.D of B}} \times 10$$

When mg% is divided by 2, m MEq/litre is obtained.

Significances

Normal level of calcium in serum ranges form 9-10.8 mg/100 ml (4.5 to 5.4 meq/l). Serum calcium level is lowered in tetany, hypopara-thyroidism, renal insufficiency, diarrhoea, rickets etc.

Calcium level is increased in hyper-parathyroidism, Vitamin D over dosage, bone tumors etc.

EXPERIMENT — 15

DETERMINATION OF DIASTASE IN URINE

Principle

The enzyme diastase, present in urine, acts upon starch and converts it into maltose.

Diastase Activity

Diastase activity is expressed as mg of starch digested by 1 ml of urine in 30 minutes at 38°C.

REAGENTS REQUIRED

1. Stach solution1 mg/ml in 0.5% sodiumchloride. Keep in a refrigerator and prepare fresh.
2. Iodine 0.02 N (0.25%)
3. Buffer solution (pH6.7);

Add 50 ml of 0.2 N potassium dihydrogen phosphate (KH$_2$ PO$_4$) and 21 ml of 0.2 N Sodium hydroxide in a volumetric flask. Dilute with water to 200 ml.

Procedure

Take ten dry test tubes and label them from 1to 10. To each of them add urine and water as shown below in the table to obtain a particular conc of urine. For tubes numbers 6 to 10 use diluted urine (1 ml urine+9ml distilled water).

To all the tubes add 2 ml of the buffer solution and 2 ml of the starch solution. Mix the contents and place all the tubes at a time in a water bath at 38°C for 30 minutes.

UNDILUTED URINE

Tube No.	Ml of Urine	Ml of water	Ml of Urine present
1.	0.5	0.5	0.5
2.	0.4	0.6	0.4
3.	0.3	0.7	0.3
4.	0.2	0.8	0.2
5.	0.1	0.9	0.1

DILUTED URINE (1 in 10)

Tube No.	Ml of Urine	Ml of water	Ml of Urine present
6.	0.9	0.1	0.09
7.	0.8	0.2	0.08
8.	0.7	0.3	0.07
9.	0.6	0.4	0.06
10.	0.5	0.5	0.05

After 30 minutes remove the tubes and immediately cool them in ice cold water. Keep the tubes in order and add iodine starting from tube no 10.

Add one drop of iodine. If blue colour appears, and fades away, pass on to the next tube. If the first drop does not give a blue colour, add more iodine drop by drop, shaking after each addition, until a permanent colour is obtained.

Calculations

If test tube No. 9 gives blue colour and tube no 8 does not which indicate that 0.07 ml of urine has digested completely 2 ml of starch in 30 minutes at 38°C.

Therefore, the amount of starch digested by 1 ml of urine under identical condition is 2/0.07=28.5 units.

Serum amylase activity can be tested by same procedure.

Significances

Normal level of urine diastase is 3-32 units. Urinary diastase activity increases to a great extent in pancreatitis.

Normal level of serum amylase activity is 5-20 units. It is raised in acute parcreatitis, intestinal obstruction and acute parotitis.

Slight elevation may occur in perforated peptic ulcers, pancreatic tumors, acute peritonitis and appendicitis. In Renal failure, serum amylase activity is increased, opioids raise the level of serum amylase. Amylase activity is decreased in liver disease.

EXPERIMENT — 16

TEST FOR LIPASE

Lipase hydrolyses fat. During the hydrolysis fatty acids are liberated.

Principle

Phenolphthalein gives pink colour in alkaline pH. In acidmedium phenolphthalein is colour-less.

REAGENTS REQUIRED

    (i) Phenolphthalein indicator
    (ii) Sodium hydroxide 0.1 N
   (iii) Milk.

Procedure

Take 2 ml of milk in a test tube. Add 1 ml of pancreatic extract and 2-3 drops of phenolphthalein solution and make the solution alkaline by adding N/10 sodium hydroxide. Incubate the tube in a water bath at 37°C. During the incubation, lipase liberates fatty acids from the fat present in milk. The pink colour slowly disappears when acids are liberated from the fat. This indicates the presence of lipase in the pancreatic extract.

ESTIMATION OF SERUM LIPASE ACTIVITY

Principle

Serum is incubated with an olive oil emulsion and the fatty acids produced is titrated with sodium hydroxide.

REAGENTS REQUIRED

1. **Gum acacia 5%** : Suspend 5 g of gum acacia in 100 ml of warm water containing 0.2 g sodium benzoate. Mix well and keep it for 12 hrs.

2. Olive oil emulsion. Homogenize a mixture of equal parts of olive oil and 5% suspension of gumacacia.

3. **Buffer solution** : Dissolve 4.7 g of anhydrous disodium phosphate (Na_2HPo_4) and 1.4 g of monopotassium phosphate (KH_2PO_4) in water, make up the volume to 100 ml.

4. **Phenolphthalein solution 1%** : Dissolve 1 g of phenolphthalein in 100 ml of 95% alcohol.

5. **Sodium hydroxide 0.05 N** : Dilute 5 ml of 1 N Sodium hydroxide to 100 ml with distilled water.

Procedure

Take two conical flasks (25ml capacity). Add 2 ml of water and 1 ml of serum into each flask. Place one flask (Marked as control) into boiling water bath for 5 minutes and cool. Then add 0.5 ml of buffer solution and 2 ml of olive oil emulsion to both flasks, shake will and incubate at 37°C for 24 hrs. Then add 3 ml of 95% alcohol and 2 drops of phenolphthalein solution. Titrate with 0.05 N Sodium hydroxide until the appearance of a persistant pink colour.

Calculation

ml of Sodium hydroxide for unknown sample	—	ml of sodium hydroxide for for control	=	Units of Lipase activity per ml of serum

Significances

The normal lipase activity is 1.5 units. Elevated level occurs in pancreatitis.

EXPERIMENT — 17

SPUTUMCULTURES

Sputum may be obtained by postural drainage or by having the patient in-hale an aerosol of warm saline. Bronchial secretions may be obtained by transtracheal aspirations.

For young children nasopharyngeal swabs should be used.

Total morning sputum specimen should be sent to the laboratory. Tubercle bacilli remain viable in refrigerated sputum, but pneumococci and haemophilus influenzae fail to survive over night refrigeration.

The laboratory should culture a number of dilutions of the sputum specimen after homogenization.

In suspected pneumonia, Gram stains of sputum may show gram positive cocci, gram negative rods (klebsiella infection) or long gram positive rods (Pulmonary anthrax). When tuberculosis is suspected, the acid-fast stain is useful. The presence of branching mycelial fragments, and yeast cells suggests a fungus infection.

EXPERIMENT — 18

EXAMINATION OF FECES

The feces include the residue remaining in the intestine after the digestion and absorption of food together with products of intestinal secretions, epithelial debris, and bacterial growth and decomposition.

Under normal conditions the consistency may vary from a thin, pasty discharge to a firmly formed stool. Stools which are very thin and watery have a pathological significance.

The normal reaction of the feces is alkaline (pH 7 to 7.5) Ingestion of large amount of lactose may cause an acid reaction.

BLOOD IN THE FECES

The detection of minute amount blood in the feces is useful in the diagnosis of certain disorders. e.g. in gastro-intestinal cancer, gastric and duodenal ulcer.

Examinations of feces for parasitism

Detection of parasites and their ova such as hookworm, tapeworm etc is of considerable importance. If the stool is firm or pasty it should be treated with water before the examination.

EXPERIMENT — 19

ROUTES OF ADMINISTRATION OF DRUGS

Intra-muscular

Drugs given by im route are absorbed more quickly than those given by subcutaneous route.

Favorite sites are the deltoid or triceps of the upper arm and the upper lateral quadrants of the buttocks. The skin should be cleaned with an antiseptic and the needle (1½ inch, 20 or 22 gauge) inserted with a quick thrust at right angles to and through the skin and into the muscle. It is essential to aspirate before finally injecting, to make sure that the needle is not in a blood vessel.

Procaine penicillin G is given by im route.

Subcutaneous

Small quantities of liquid medicament can be given by subcutaneous route. Subcutaneous injection is given by pinching up the skin, previously cleaned with an antiseptic (e.g. alcohol), between thumb and fore finger and then firmly and quickly inserting the needle through all layers of the skin. The solution is injected with ease if the point of the needle (22 no) has penetrated into the subcutaneous tissues and is not lodged in skin or muscle. The sites of subcutaneous administration are the extensor surfaces of the upper arms, the back, and the lateral aspects of the thighs. Steroid hormones are given by subcutaneous route.

Intravenous route

Injection of fluids by vein is useful when rapid absorption of the drug is desired and when fluid cannot be taken by mouth.

the sites of intravenous administration are the veins of the forearm and dorsam of the hand.

The site of injection should be cleaned with an antiseptic and the limb placed in comfortable position to minimize movement. The veins are distended bycuff. Before inserting the needle, all air is removed from the tubing, in order to avoid air embolism.

Dextrose solution is given through iv route. I.V. fluid administration can fail because of not having the needle in the lumen of the vein, an obstruction in the needle, allowing the bevel of the needle to rest too firmly against the inside of the vein wall or proximal venous thrombosis.

Extravasation of fluid or blood into the tissues is a common complication, due to faulty veinpuncture or displacment of the needle, and causes swelling and pain at the site of injection. Acid solution, alkaline solution and hypertonic solution produce severe pain. In such situation it is important to remove the needle immediately. The area should be massaged so as to disperse the fluid more rapidly. The area may be infiltrated with physiologic saline or water to dilute the irritant.

When it is impossible to locate a vein, it is necessary to perform a vein cut-down and cannulize a vein. This situation arise when a patient is in shock and all normally accesible veins are collapsed or in the obese or in the very young. This is also useful when large amounts of fluids must be given within a short period of time.

EXPERIMENT — 20

URINE ANALYSIS

The urine is the main excretary fluid eliminated through the agency of kidney. Most of the waste products are excreted through urine. Urine contains a large number of inorganic and organic substances. Any sample of Normal urine. contains a few substances which are called Normal constituents.

In pathological condition some substances are present in addition which are called as Abnormal constituents.

Collection of Urine

For quantitative analysis 24 hrs sample is used. 10 ml toluene is added as preservative. Quantity of urine excreted per day is 1000-1500 ml. Normal human Urine is straw in colour.

Specific gravity lies between 1.012 to 1.024.

Analysis of normal constituents of urine

Analysis of inorganic constituents.

  (i) **Test for chloride :** To 3 mlof urine add 1 ml of conc nitric acid (to prevent the precipitation of urates by silver nitrate) and 1 ml of silver nitrate. A white precipitate of silver chloride indicates the presence of chlorides in urine.

 (ii) **Test for sulphate :** To 2 ml of urine add 0.55 ml of conc hydrochloric acid and 2 mlof barium chloride. A white precipitate indicates the formation of baruim sulphate.

(iii) **Test for phosphorus:** To 5 ml of urine add 5 drops of conc nitric acid and a little ammonium molybdate and warm. Canary yellow precipitate of ammonium phosphmolybdate is formed.

 (iv) **Test for calcium :** To 5 ml of urine add 1 ml of strong ammonia. Boil. Filter and wash the residue with water.

Dissolve the precipitate in 5 drops of acetic acid and add 1 ml of potassium oxalate solution (2%). A white precipitate of calcium oxalate indicates the presence of calcium.

(v) **Test for ammonia :** To 5 ml of urine add 2 % sodium carbonate till the solution is alkaline to litmus. (Red papers turns blue) Boil. Hold piece of moistened red litmus paper at the mouth of the tube. Red litmus turns blue by the liberated ammonia.

Analysis of organic Constituents

(i) To 2 ml of urine add 5 drops of sodium hypobromite reagent (100 ml of 40% NaOH containing 10 ml liquid bromine).
Brick effervescence of nitrogen occurs.

(ii) **Test for uric acid :** To 2 ml of urine add a few drops of phosphotungstic acid reagent and a few drops of 20% Na_2Co_3. Appearance of blue colour indicates the presence of uric acid.

(iii) **Test for Creatinine :** Take 2 ml of urine in a test tube Add 2 ml of picric acid followed by few drops of sodium hydroxide. Reddish brown colour indicates the presence of creatinine.

(iv) **Test for Urobilinogen :** To 5 ml of urine add 1ml of Ehrlich's reagent (Ehrlich reagent consists of 0.7g of p-dimethyl aminobenzaldehyde in 100 ml of water with 150 ml of concentrated hydrochloric acid).
Mix well and keep it for 5 minutes. A red colour is seen when viewed through the mouth of the test tube.

EXPERIMENT — 21

ANALYSIS OF ABNORMAL CONSTITUENTS OF URINE

Abnormal constituents are present in urine during pathological conditions.

In diabetes mellitus, glucose is excreted through urine.

In kidney disease like nephritis, albumin is present in urine.

In hematuria and hemoglobinuria blood occurs in urine.

Bilirubin is found in urine during jaundice.

1. Test for albumin

Take 10 ml of urine in a test tube. Hold it over a flame in a slanting position for 2 minutes. Turbidity occurs, which is due to the presence of phosphate, carbonate or albumin. Add 5 drops of 10% acetic acid. If the turbidity disappears after acidification, then the turbidity is due to phosphate and carbonate. If turbidity does not disappear it indicates that albumin is present in the urine.

2. Test for glucose

To 5 ml of Benedict's reagent add 8 drops of urine. Boil for 1 to 2 minutes. A light green colour indicates 0.5% glucose, a yellow colour 1% and brick red colour 2% glucose.

3. Test for ketone bodies

Rothera's test for acetone : To 5 ml of urine add enough solid ammonium sulphate to saturate it completely and to leave some solid undissolved. Then 2-3 drops of nitroprusside 5% solution (fresh). Mix well and add 1 ml of strong ammonium hydroxide dropwise along the side. Keep it for 10 minutes. Development of purple coloured (permanganate coloured) ring indicates the presence of acetone bodies.

4. Gerhardt's test for acetoacetic acid

To 3 ml of urine add ferric chloride solution (10%) drop. by drop until no further precipitate is formed. Filter the ferric phosphate formed. To the filtrate add ferric chloride.

A port-wine colour (Bordeaux-red colour) indicates the presence of acetoacetic acid.

5. Test for bile salts

Hay's sulphur flower test : Take 2 ml of urine in a wide test tube and sprinkle fine sulphur powder observe without mixing. The presence of bile salts is indicated by the rapid sinking of sulphur flowers to the bottom. Because bile salts decrease the surface tension.

6. Test for bilirubin

Foucher's test : To 10 ml of urine in a test tube add 5 ml of barium chloride (10% solution) and 3 drops of saturated magnesium sulphate soluion. Mix well. Barium sulphate is precipitated. After 5 minutes, filter the solution. Unfold the filter paper over one or two filter papers. Add few drops of Foucher's reagent (Foucher's reagent. Consists of 10 ml of 10% ferric chloride with 100 ml of 25% trichloracetic acid). Wet barium sulphate adsorbs yellow bilirubin. Foucher's reagent oxidises bilirubin to green biliverdin.

7. Test for blood

Benzidine test : To 3 drops of benzidine solution (12% in glacialacetic acid) Add 2 drops of hydrogen Peroxide. Add 1 drop of this to 2 ml of urine in a test tube. A blue or green colour indicate the presence of blood.

INDEX